SABINA'S CELIAC STORY

by Neva Ryan
illustrated by Behnaz Hajielyasi

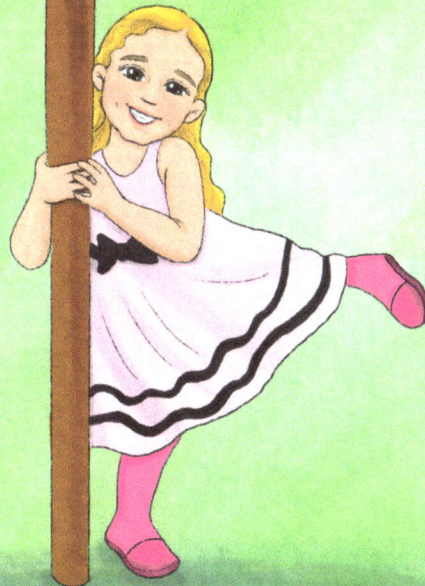

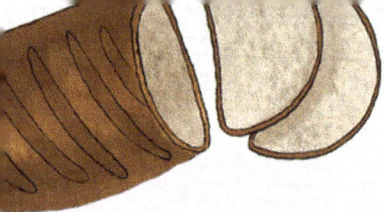

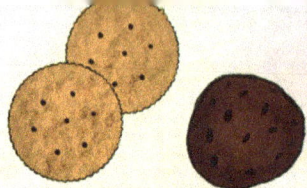

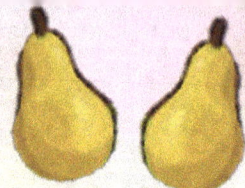

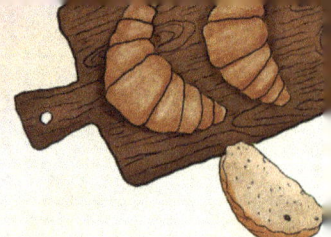

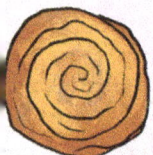

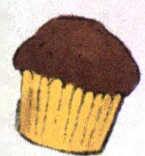

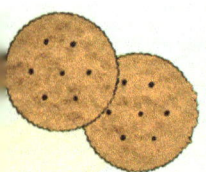

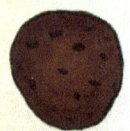

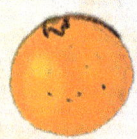

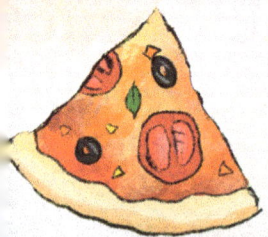

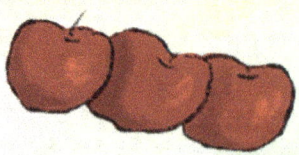

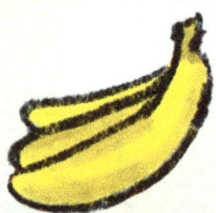

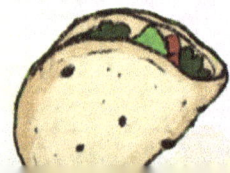

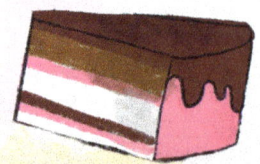

neva ryan books
Chicago, Illinois
www.nevaryanbooks.com

Library of Congress Control Number: 2022917240
ISBN 979-8-9853658-4-9 (hardcover)
ISBN 979-8-9853658-3-2 (paperback)

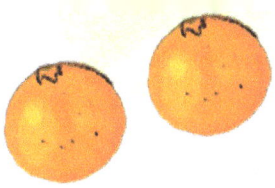

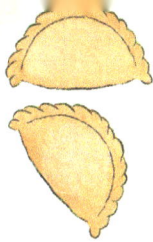

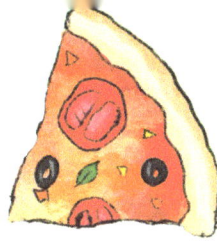

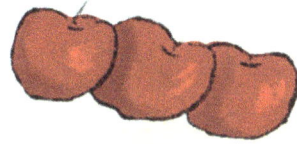

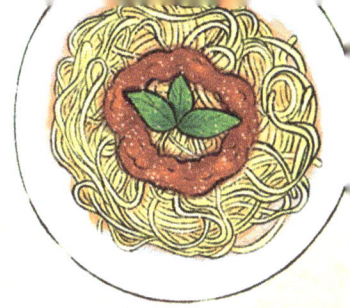

For Sabina and Olivia
and all kids everywhere with celiac disease, allergies,
or any type of dietary restriction
-N.R.

For the children of my home country of Iran
who I hope will one day know peace and freedom
-B.H.

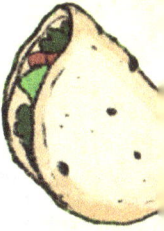

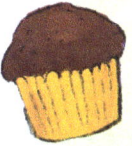

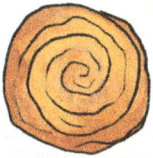

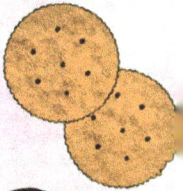

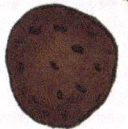

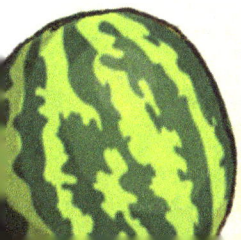

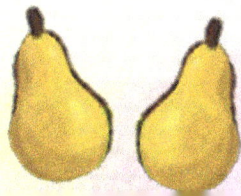

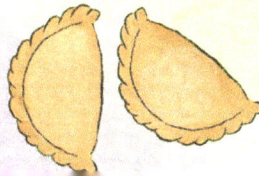

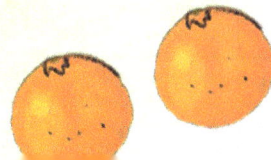

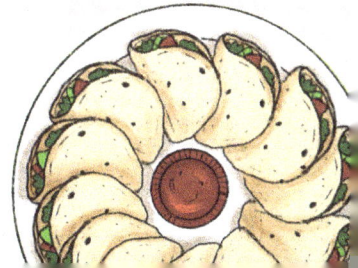

Meet Sabina, a carefree and happy child.

She's thoughtful, funny, and impeccably styled.

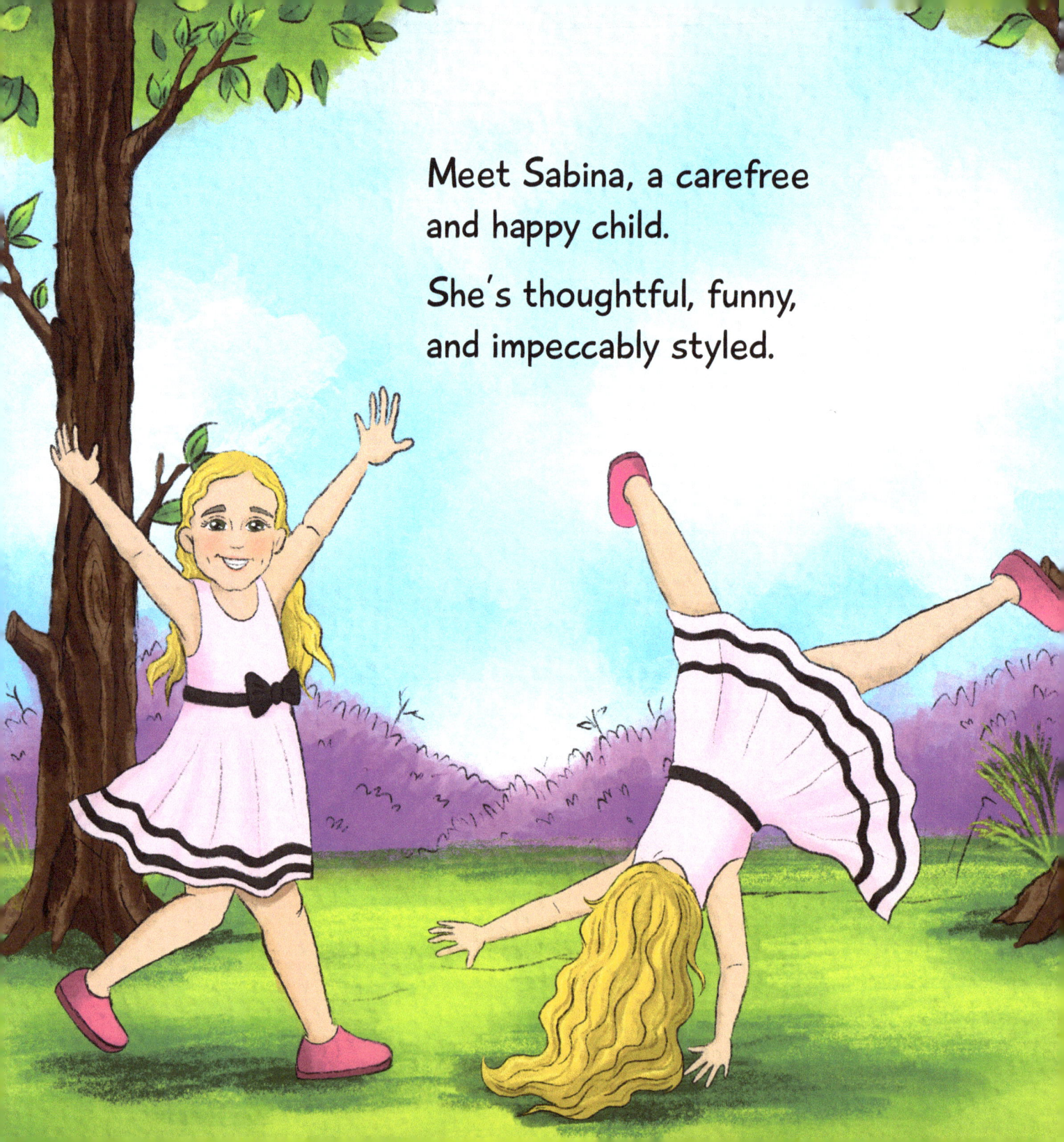

She loves to sing and dance
and cartwheel around.

When Sabina's near,
fun and laughter abound!

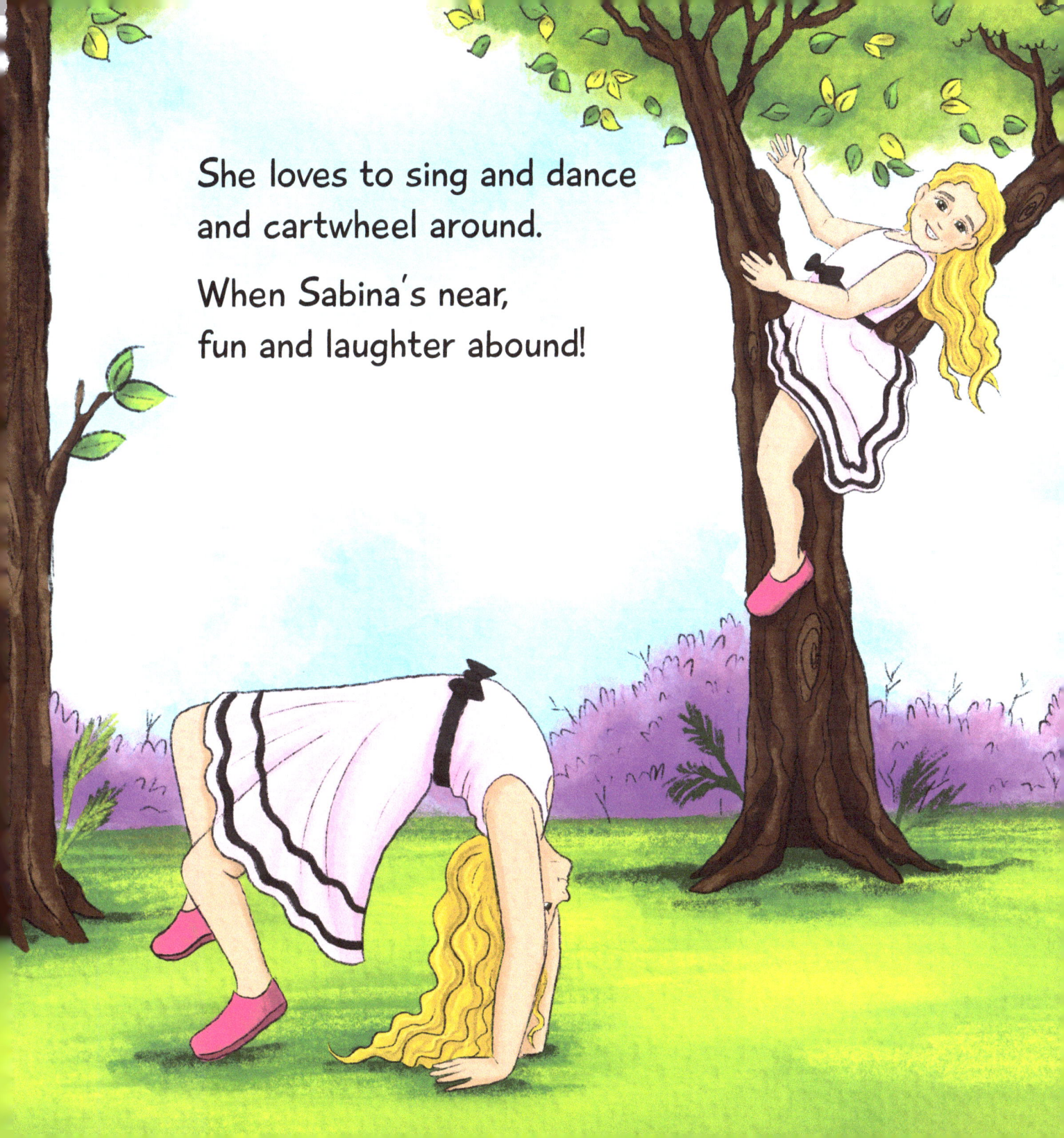

When Sabina was small, she ate dirt and sand.
For most of us, that would taste gritty and bland.
But she said that sand tasted just like honey.
Dirt was like chocolate—now that sounded funny.

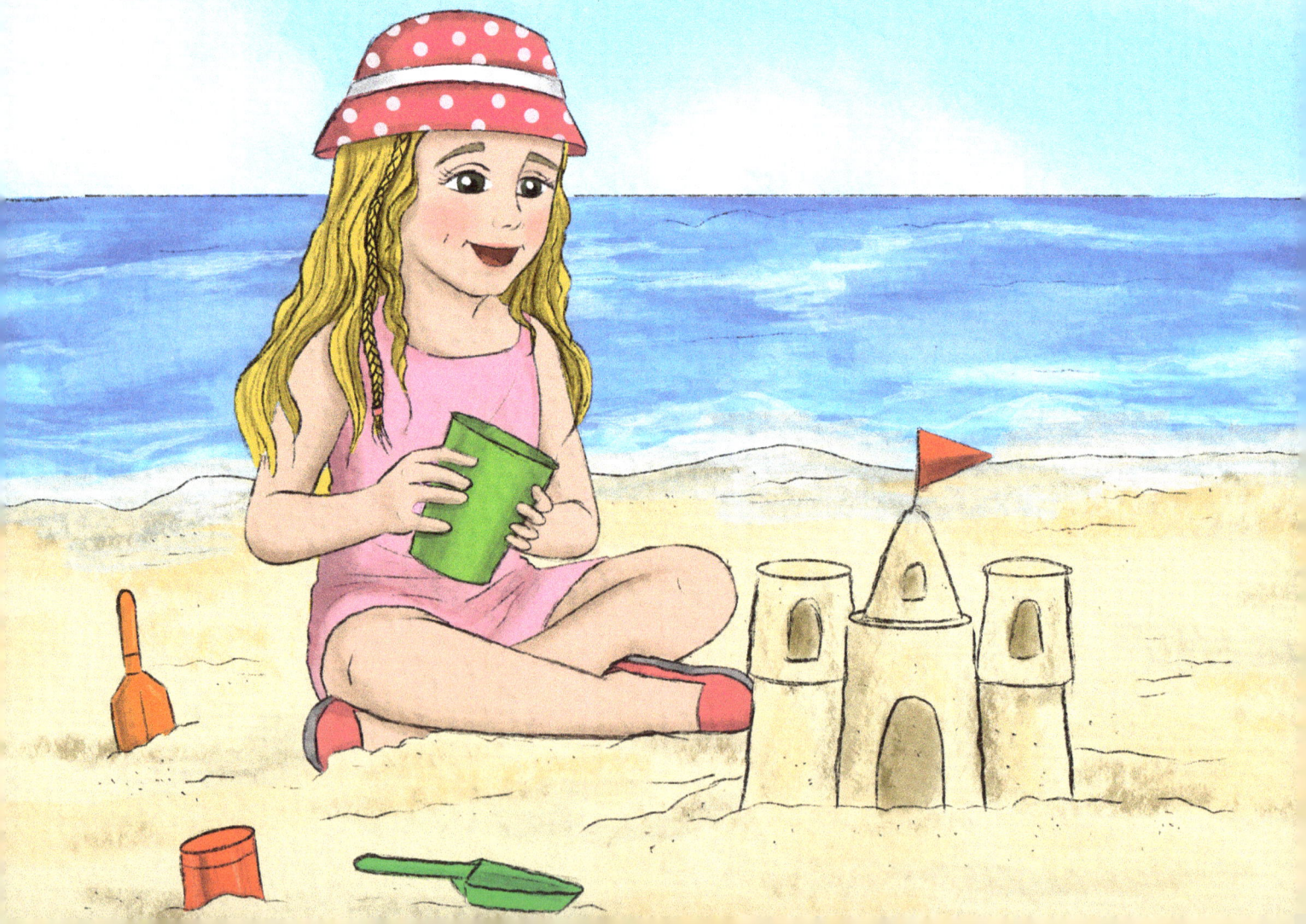

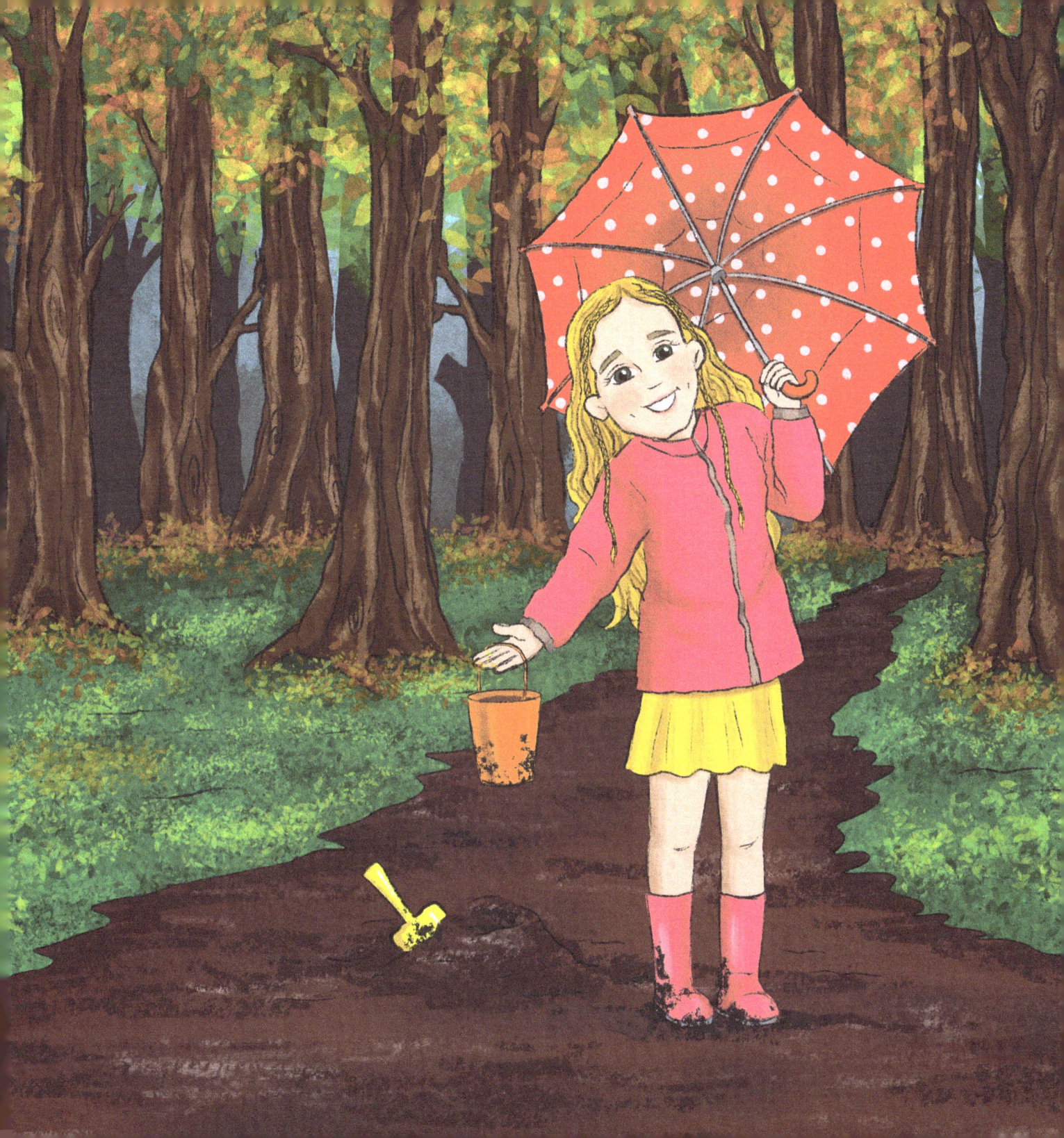

It turned out her levels of iron were low.
Iron supplements helped, but she didn't know...
That was a symptom of celiac disease,
And her body was calling out, "Help me, please!"

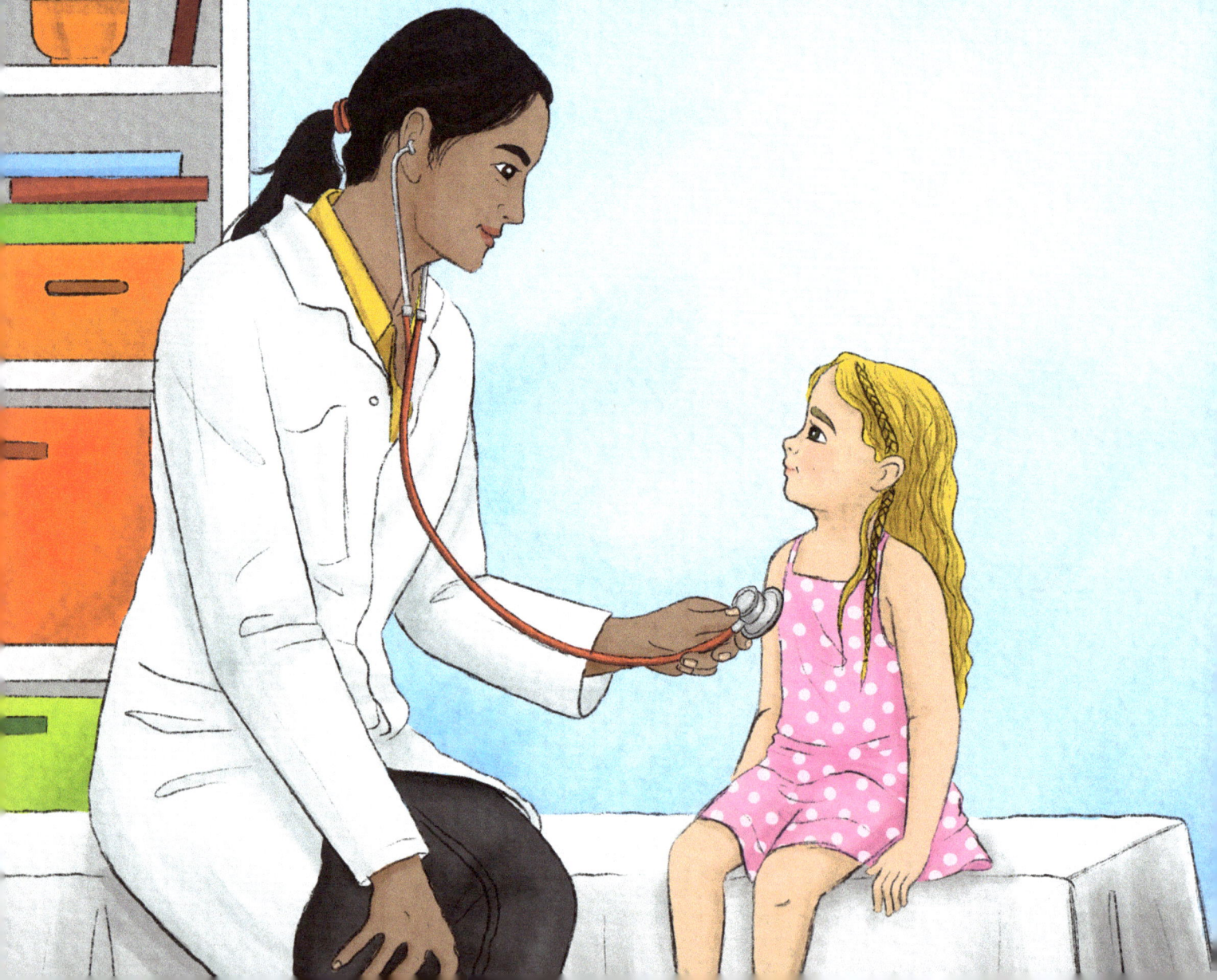

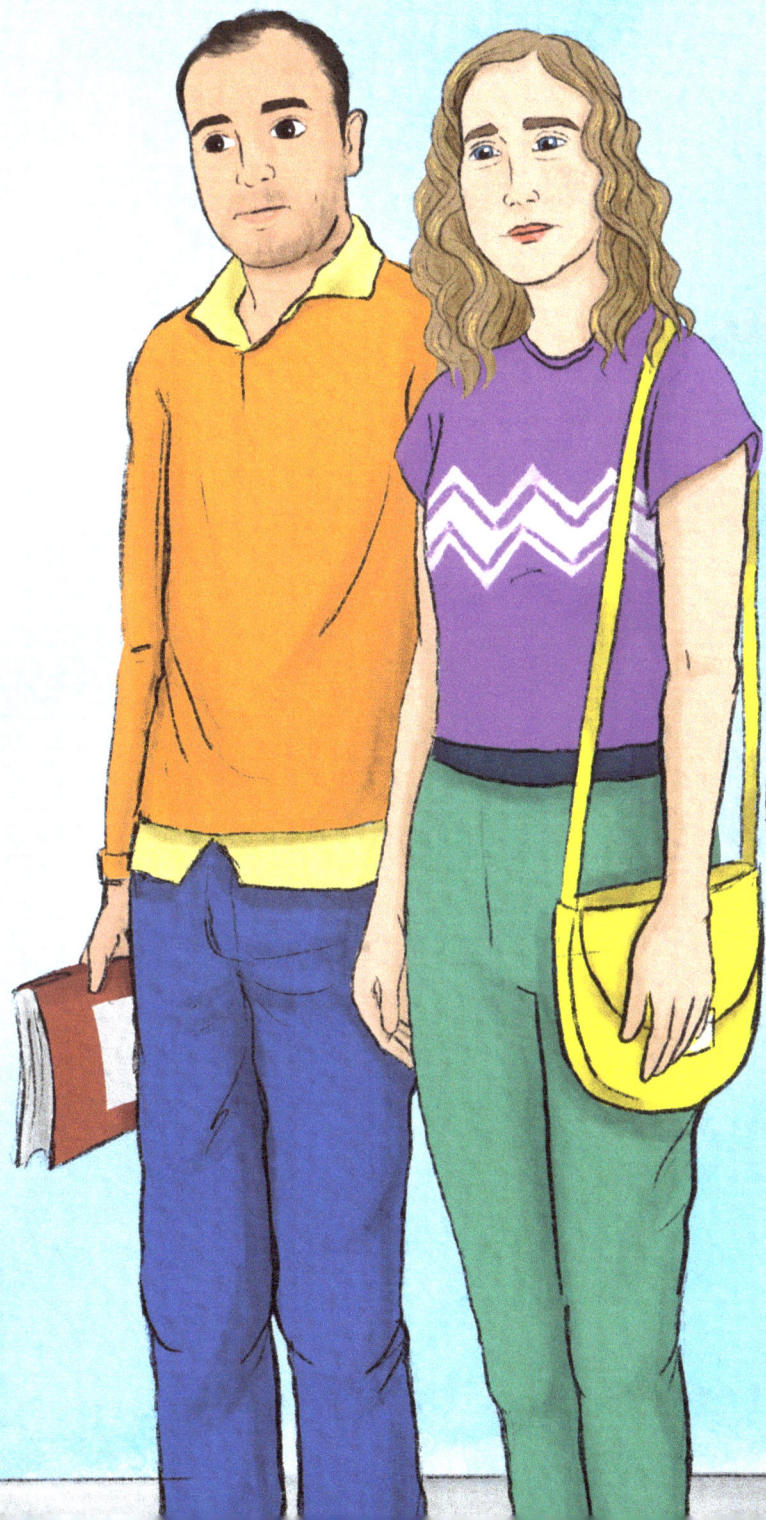

On special occasions, Sabina got sick.
Vomiting and diarrhea came on quick!
It turns out that gluten plus sugar and fat
Make the symptoms worse, but she didn't know that.

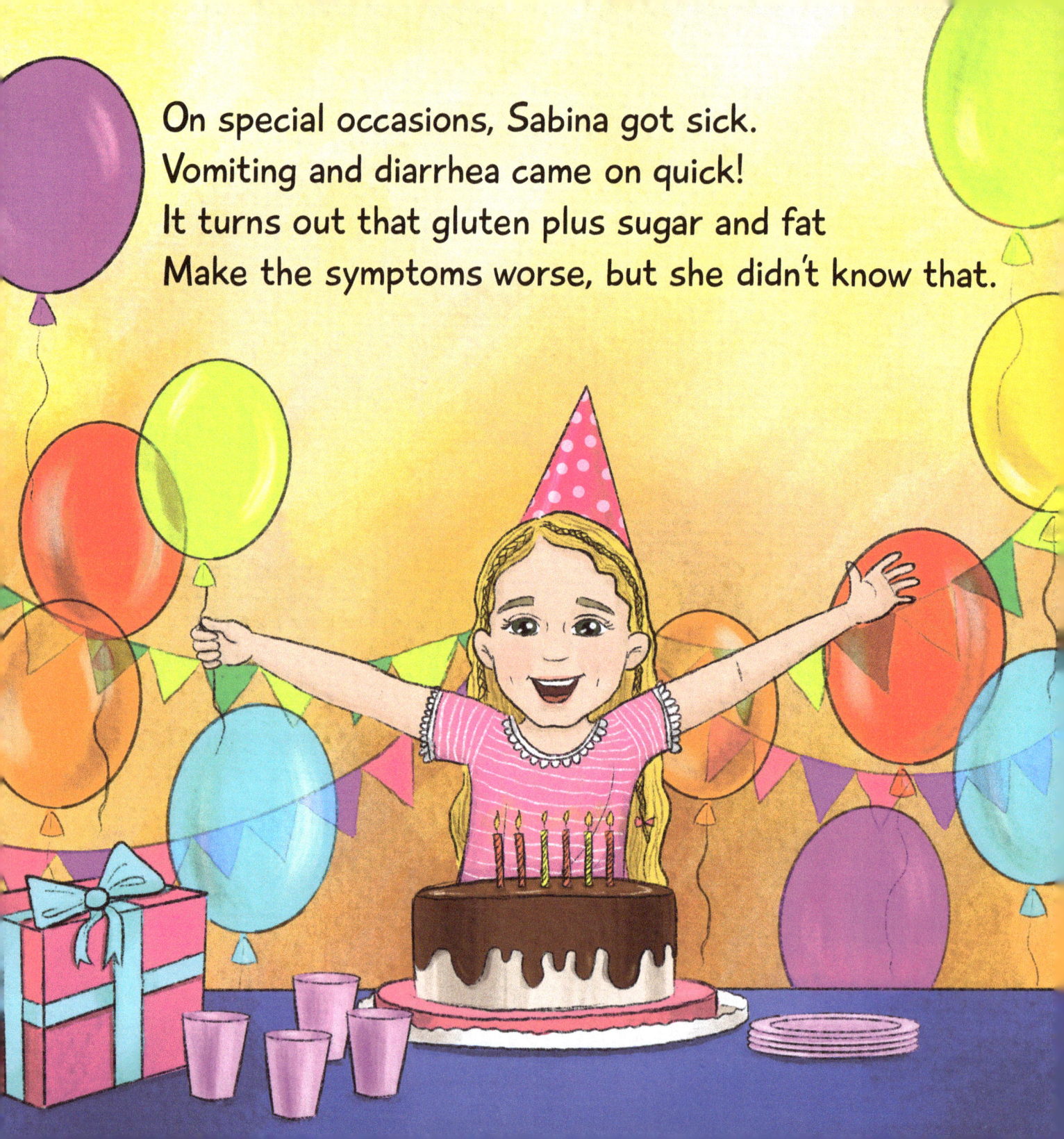

She ate lots of cookies one time on a trip
And threw up all night—that should have been a tip.
She stayed in bed the next day and missed the fun.
What could be wrong? It just baffled everyone!

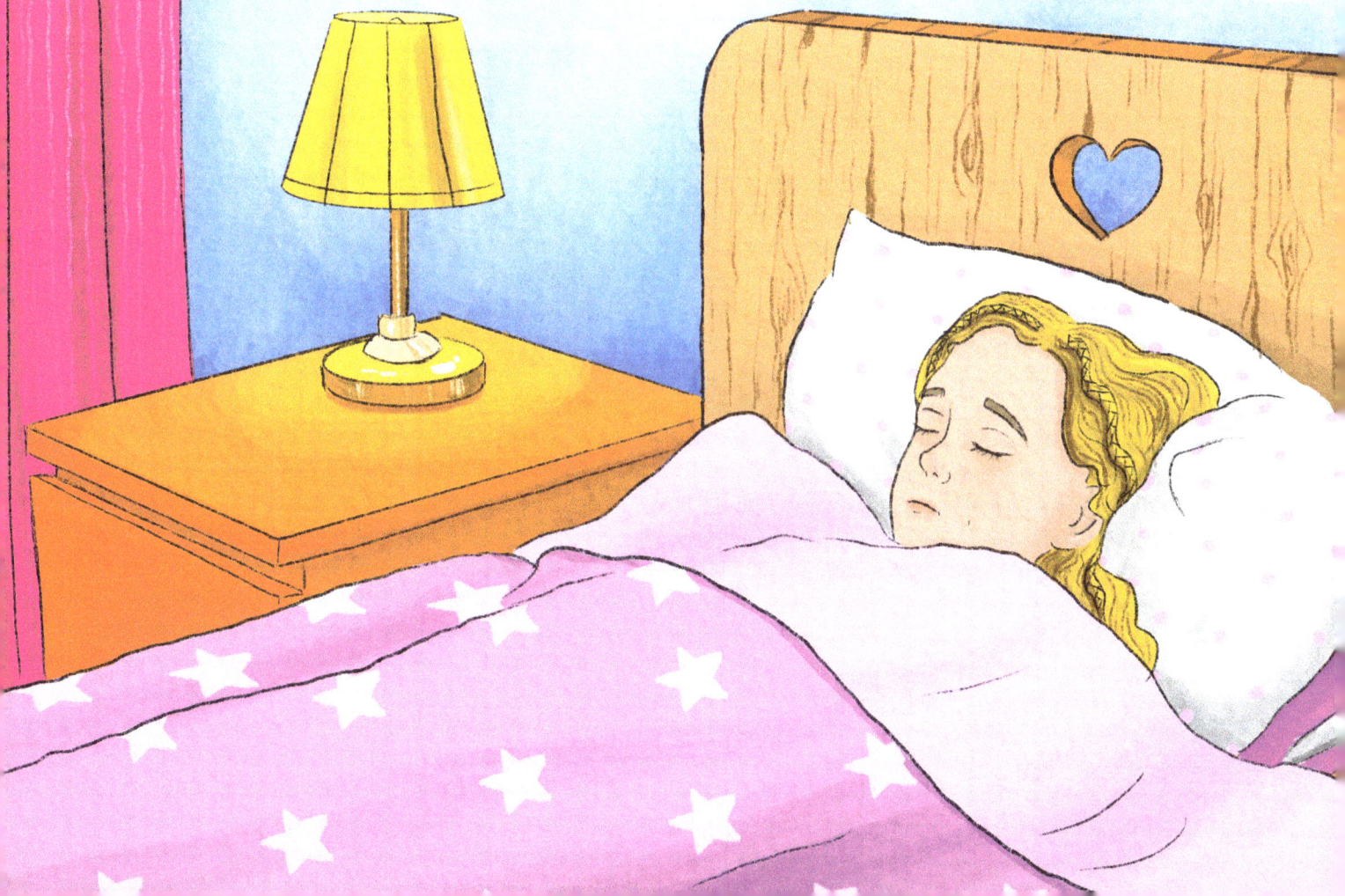

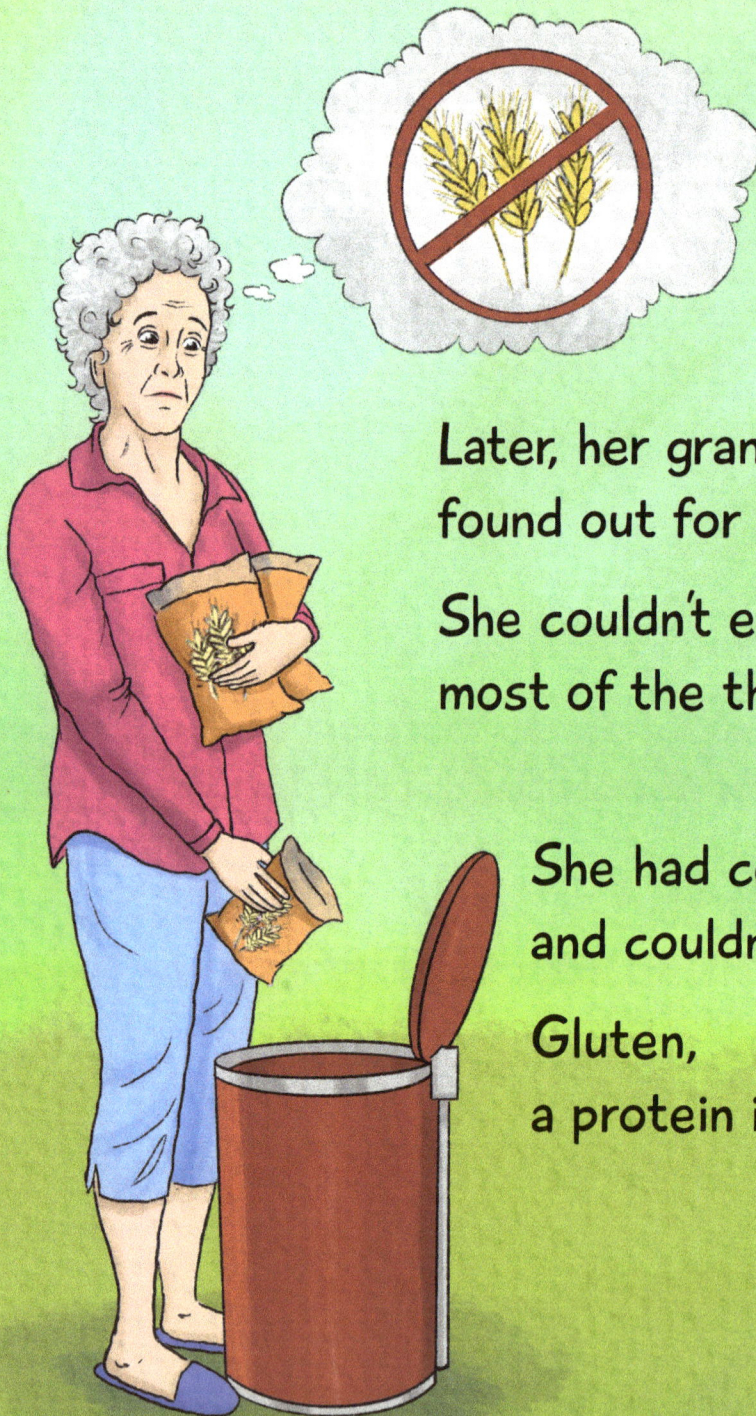

Later, her grandmother
found out for herself

She couldn't eat
most of the things on her shelf!

She had celiac disease
and couldn't eat...

Gluten,
a protein in rye, barley, and wheat.

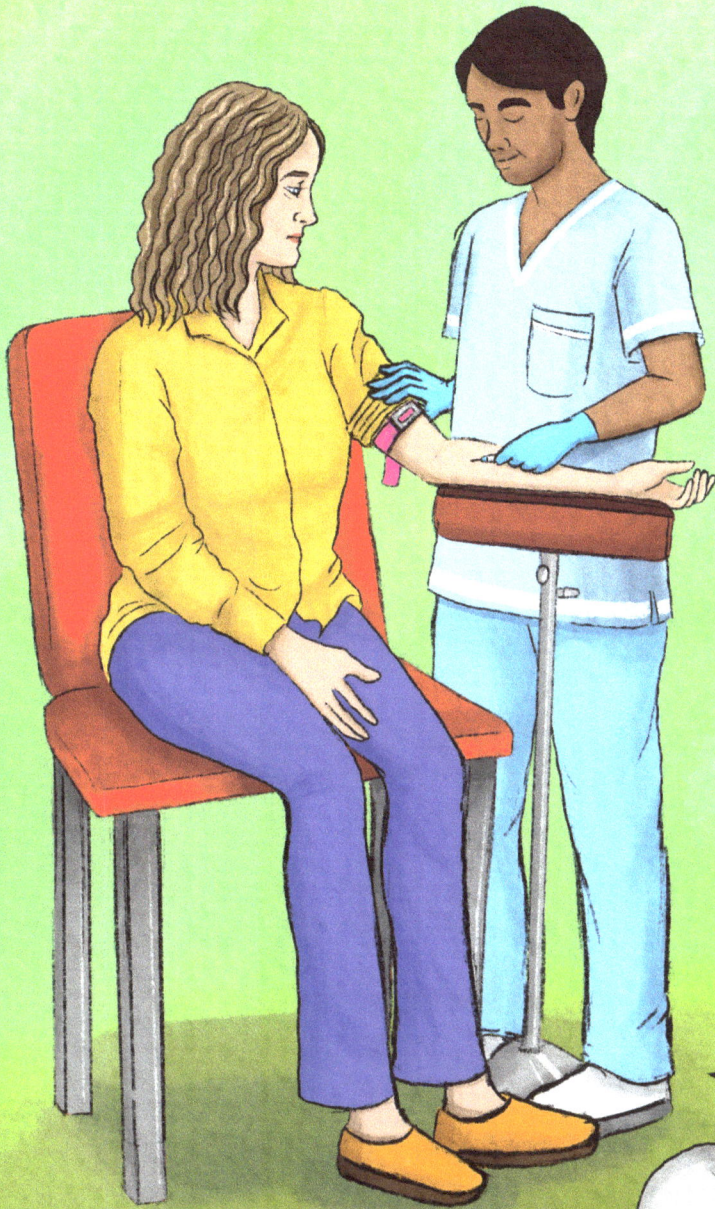

Sabina's mom got tested,
and she found out

She was a celiac, too—
without a doubt.

Sabina's turn came next
to get a blood test,

And just how it turned out,
you've probably guessed.

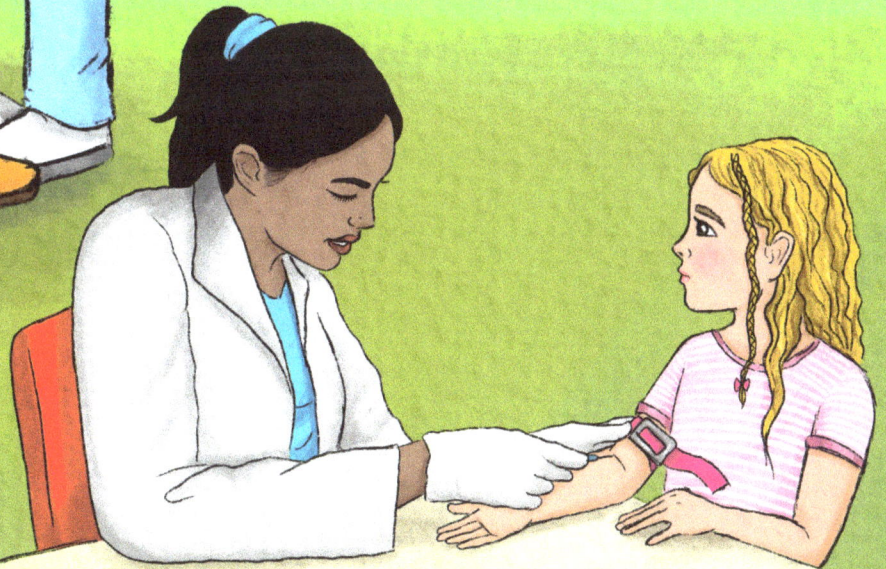

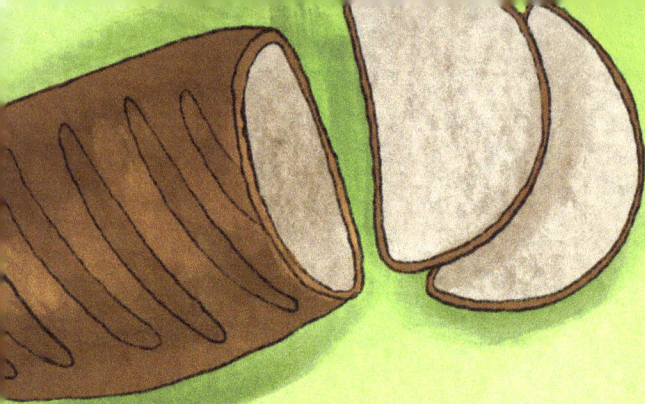

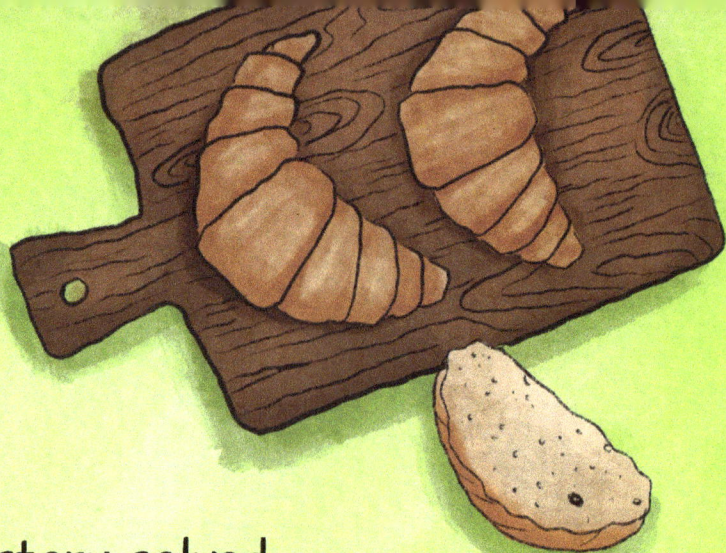

She had celiac disease—mystery solved.
Now how would she treat it? Just what was involved?

Her body could heal itself,
just as it should

If she stopped eating gluten
right then... for good.

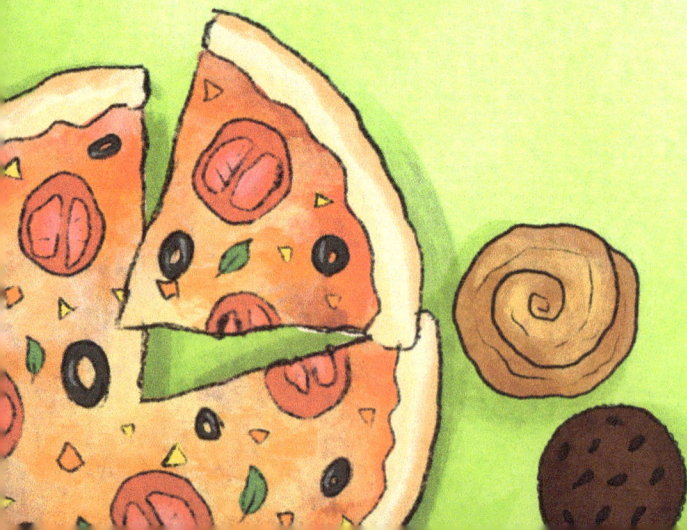

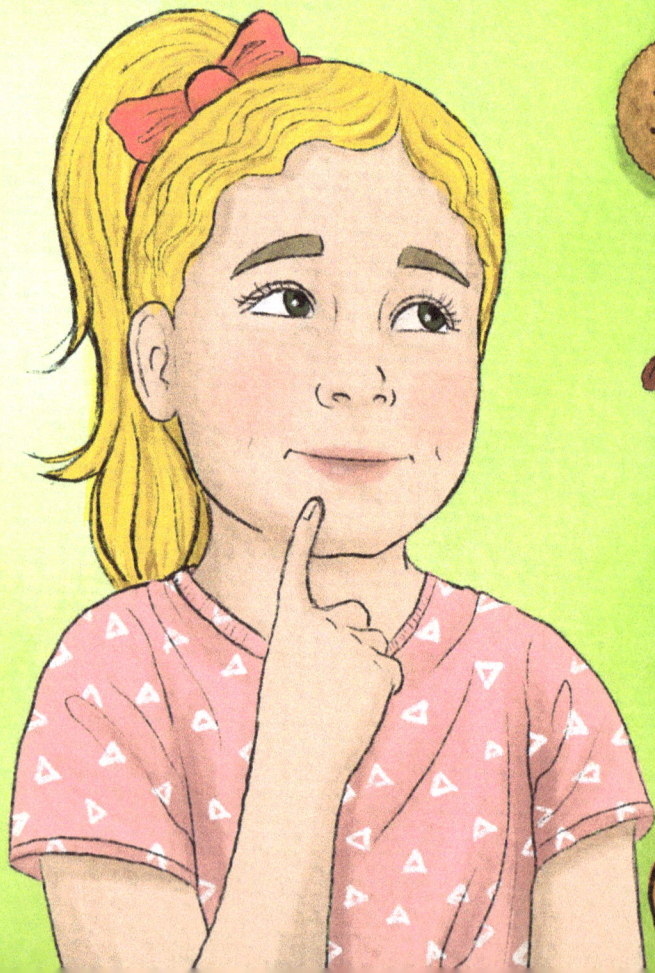

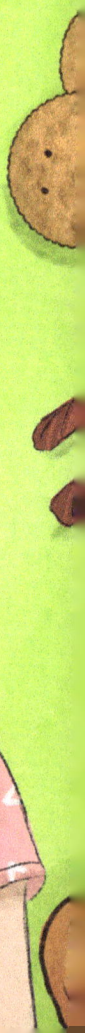

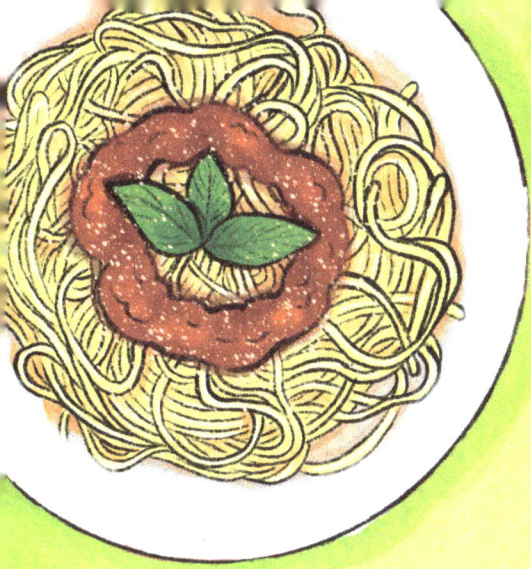

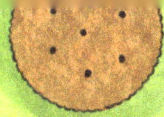

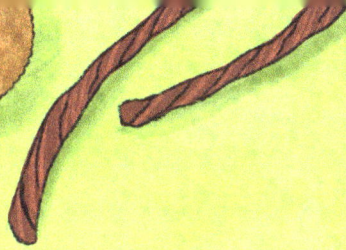

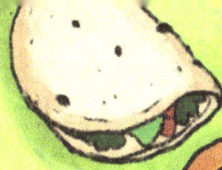

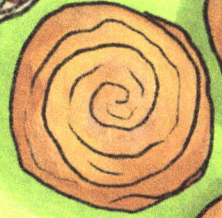

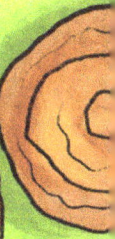

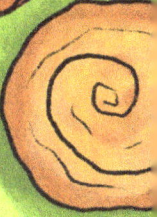

But that gluten is sneaky, she soon found out.
It's in so many foods, just lurking about.
Gluten is in bread and in pasta and cake.
It's in crackers, candy, and cookies we bake.

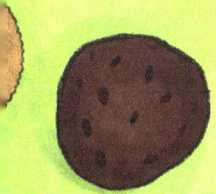

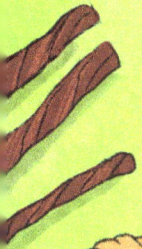

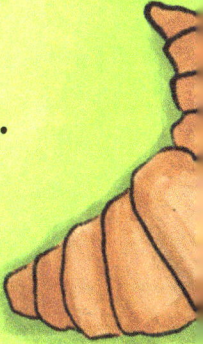

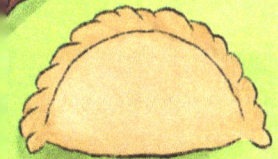

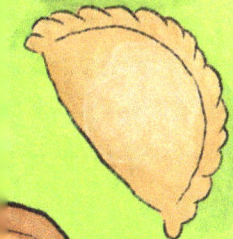

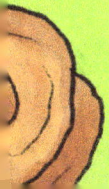

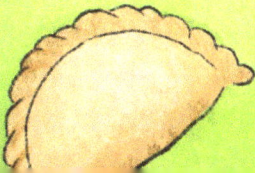

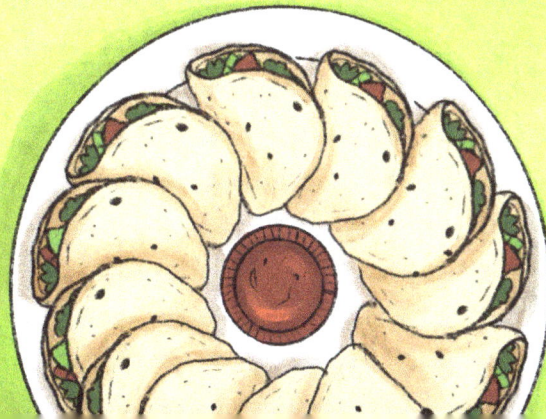

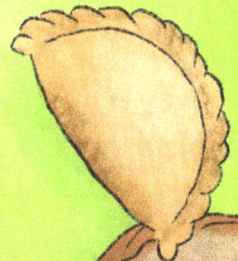

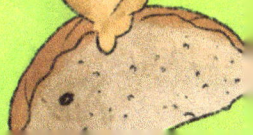

The whole family searched for gluten-free stuff,
But shopping took longer. At first it was tough!
For some foods, they didn't know what to expect.
Gluten's even in foods they didn't suspect.

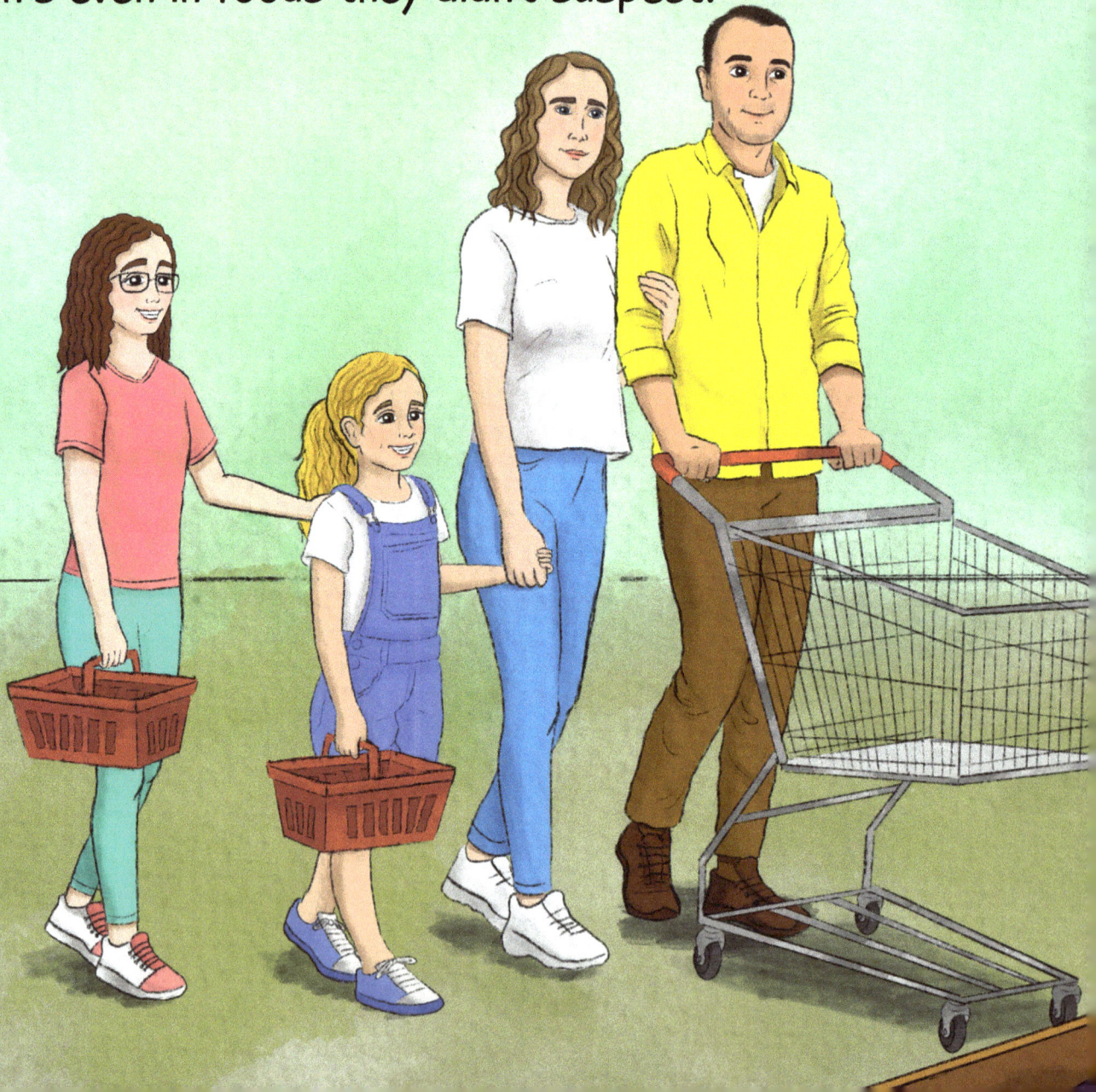

Fruit, veggies, and quinoa are all gluten free.
So are milk, eggs, and rice—easy as can be!
For the rest, they researched and checked each label
And purchased safe foods to put on their table.

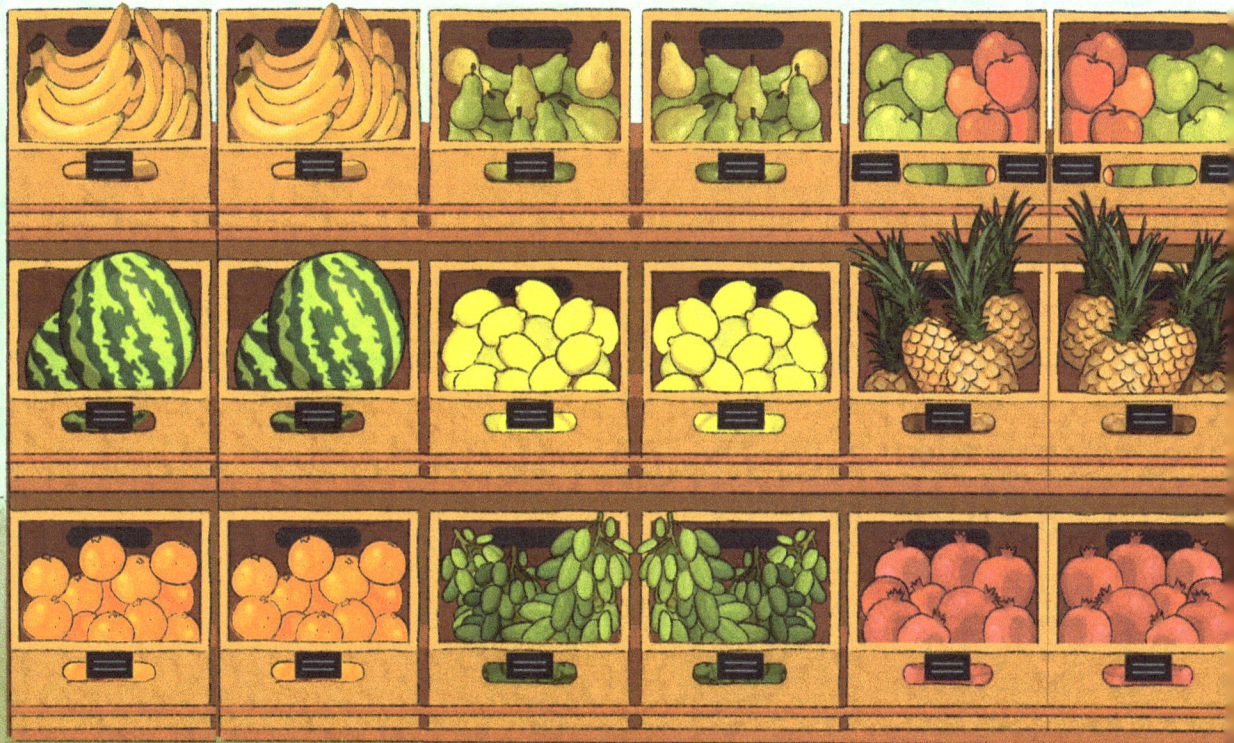

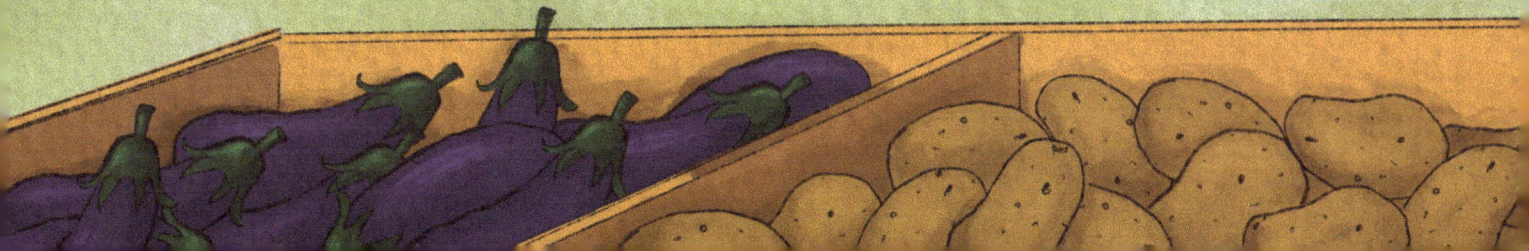

They found flour to use that didn't have wheat
For pancakes and waffles and sweet treats to eat!

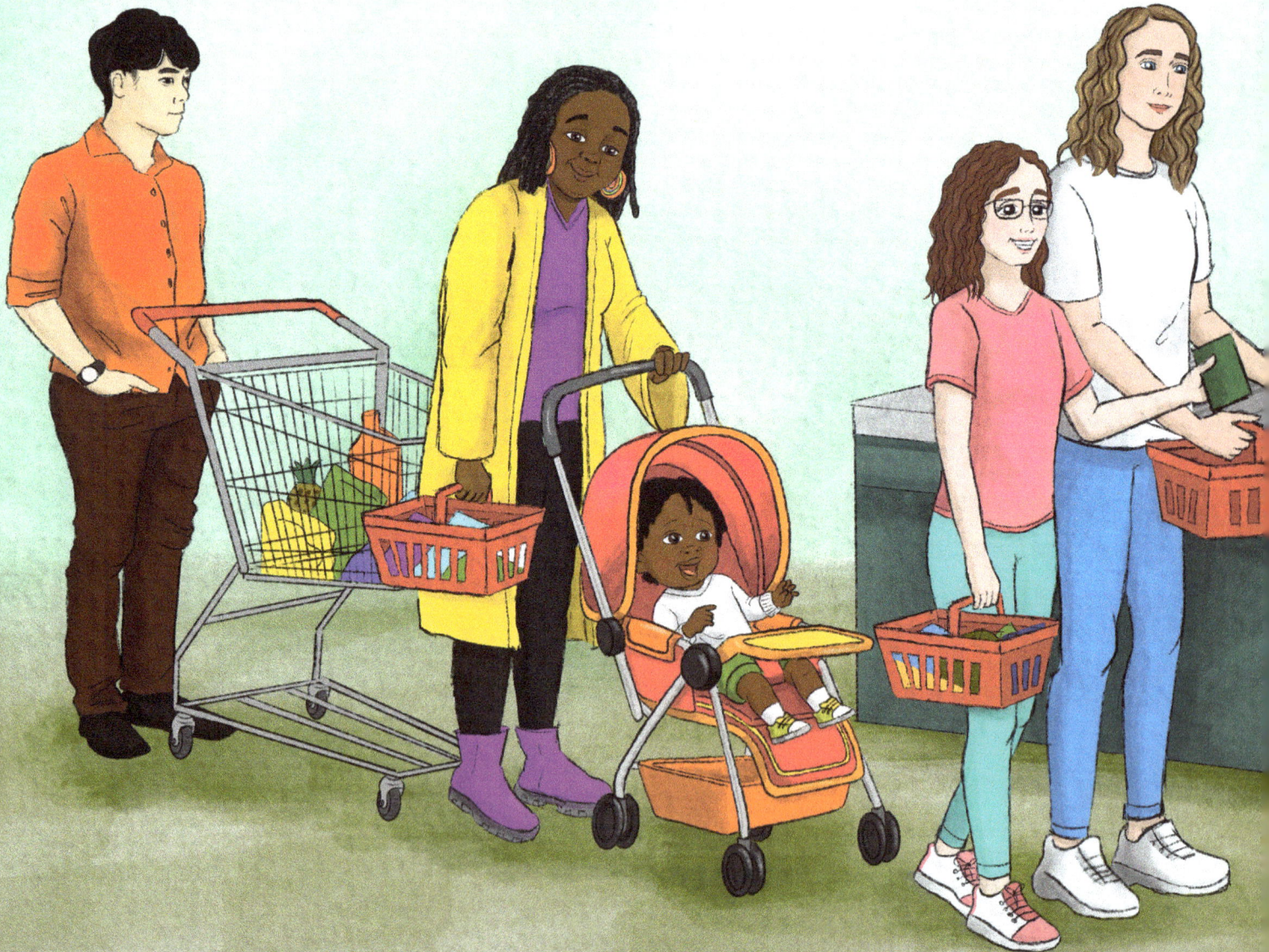

They found gluten-free pasta and crackers, too!
They found gluten-free pizza and gum to chew!

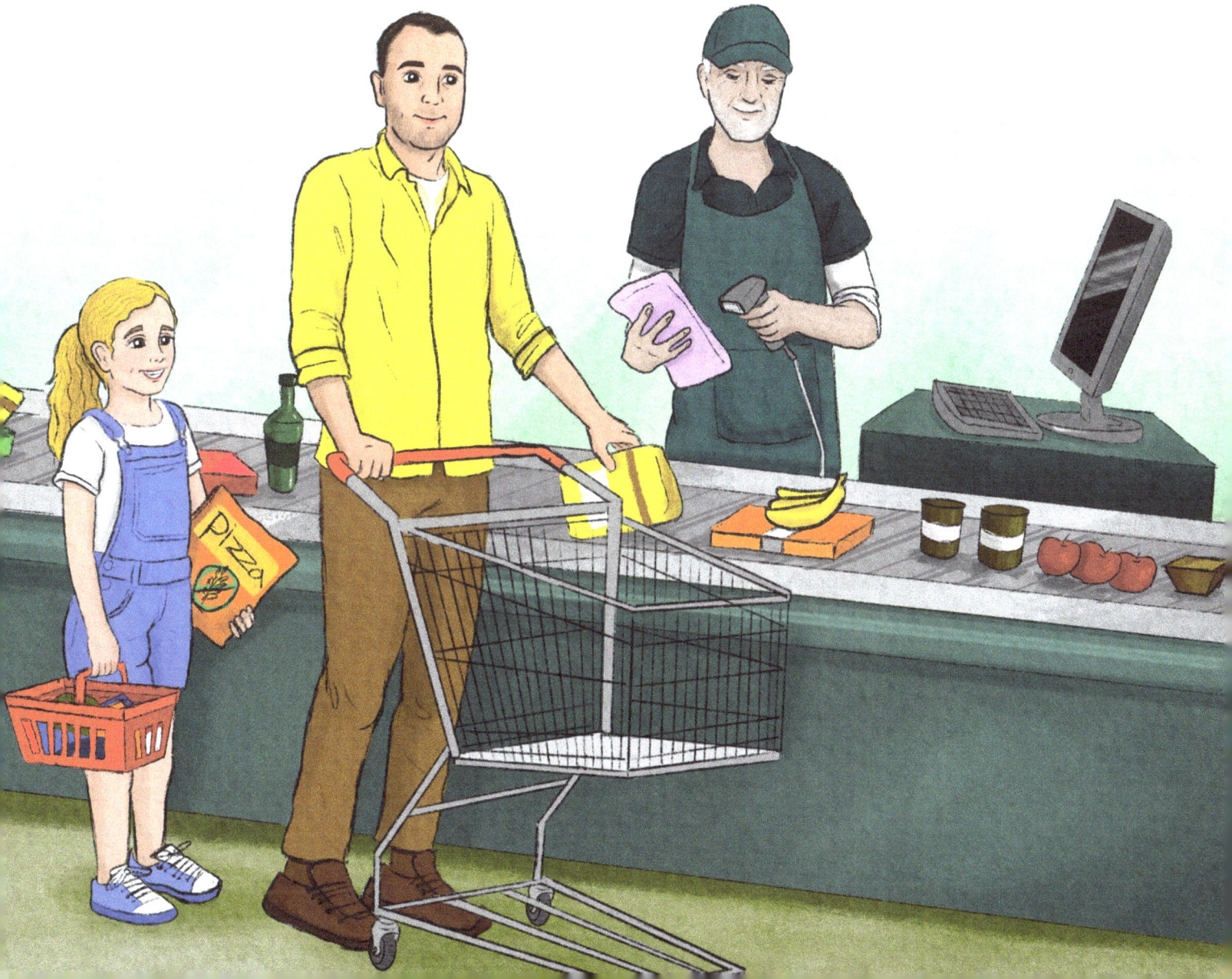

Next on the list was to clean out the kitchen.
All hands on deck—the whole fam had to pitch in!
Some things couldn't be cleaned and just had to go...
Like old spatulas used to mix cookie dough.

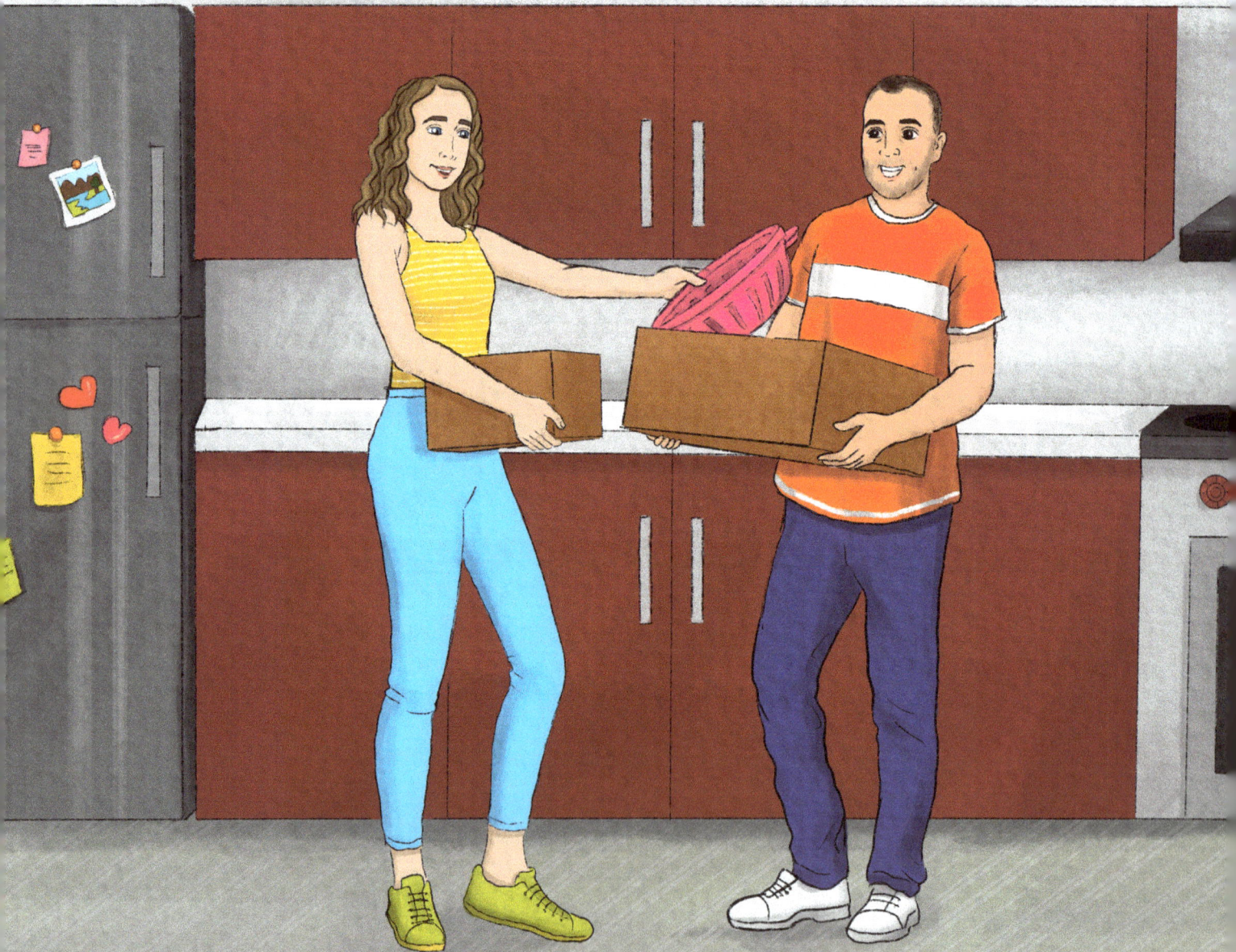

They gave away food, wooden spoons, plastic bowls,
And colanders with gluten stuck in the holes.
They replaced those things and swept every crumb up...
They washed pots and pans and each plate and each cup.

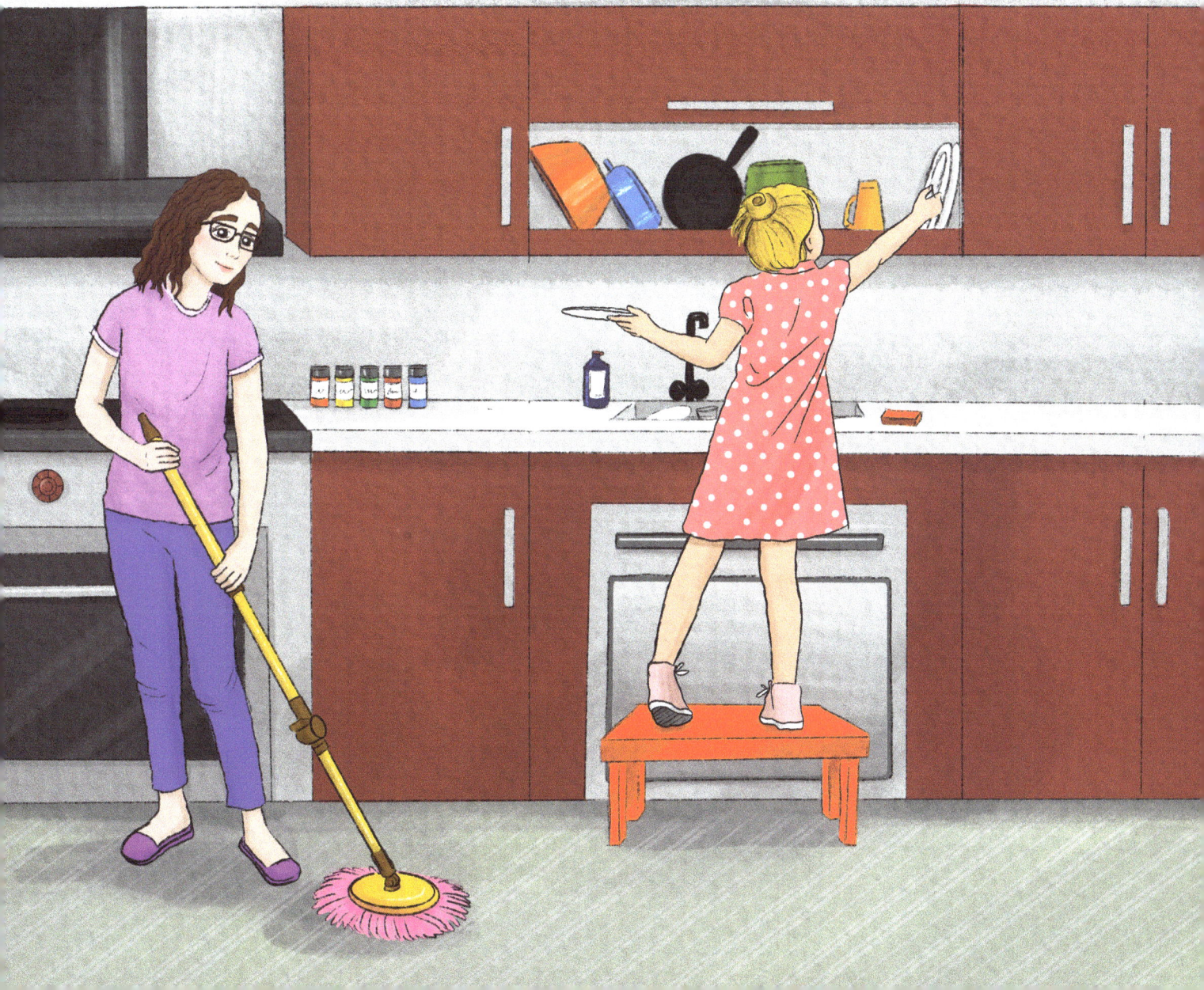

Finally, their kitchen was all gluten free,
And once more, mealtime filled Sabina with glee!
Like before, she could choose any food in sight.
At home, she felt eating suited her just right.

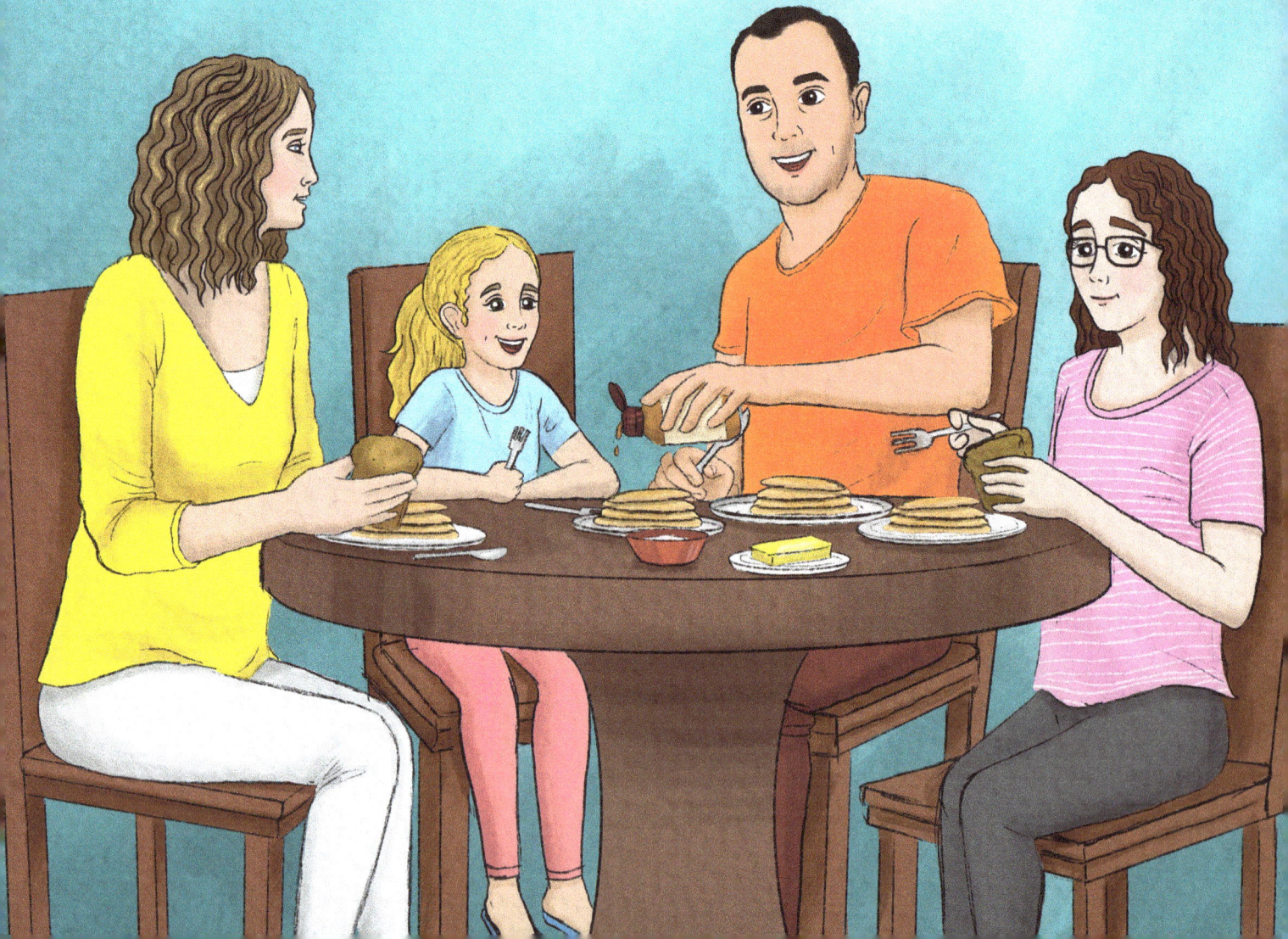

But restaurants are tricky since not all know
That if you're not careful, gluten crumbs can blow.
One crumb of gluten can make Sabina sick;
So, she must be sure there's safe food she can pick.

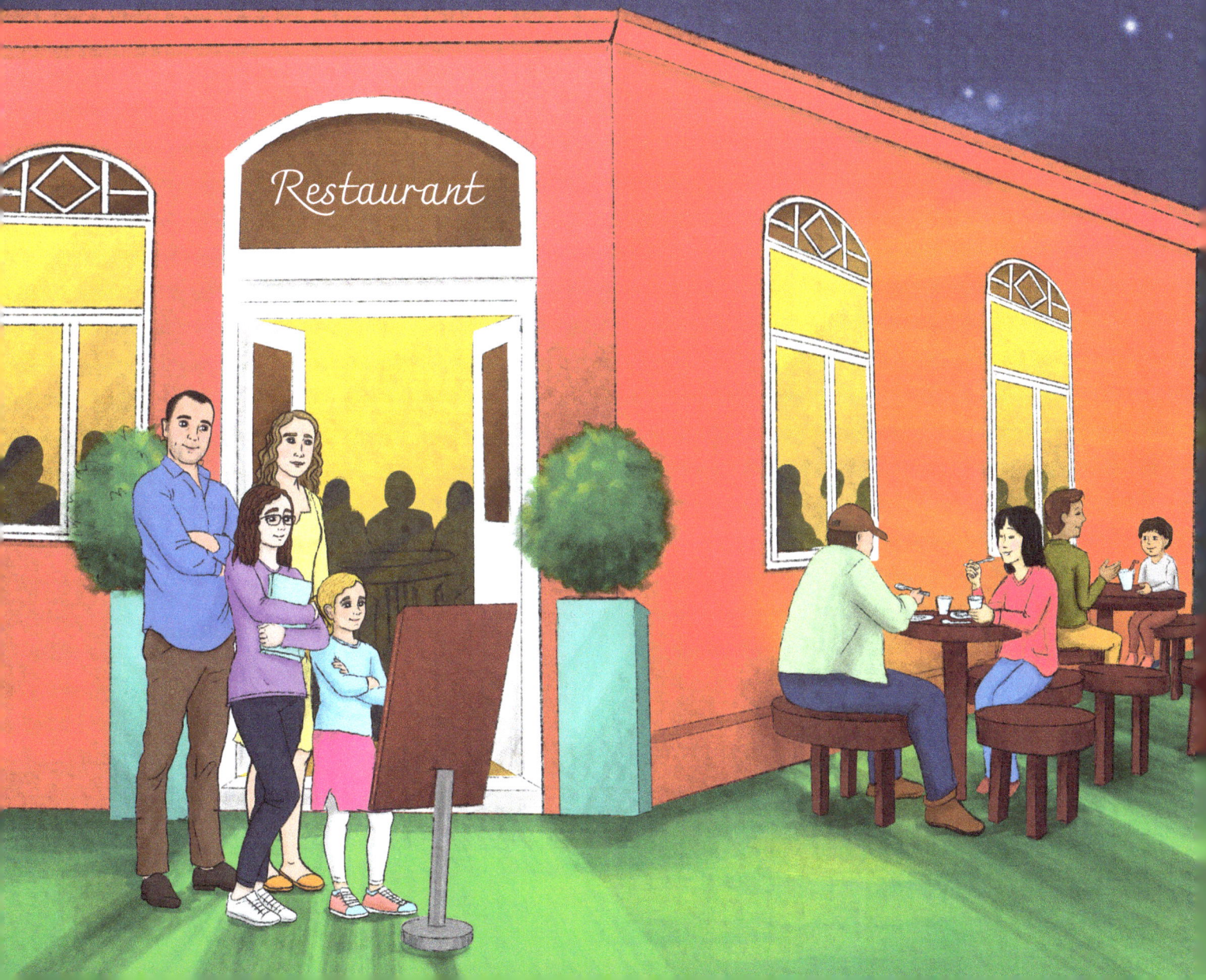

It's also quite hard to miss out on a treat,
Especially one Sabina loves to eat.

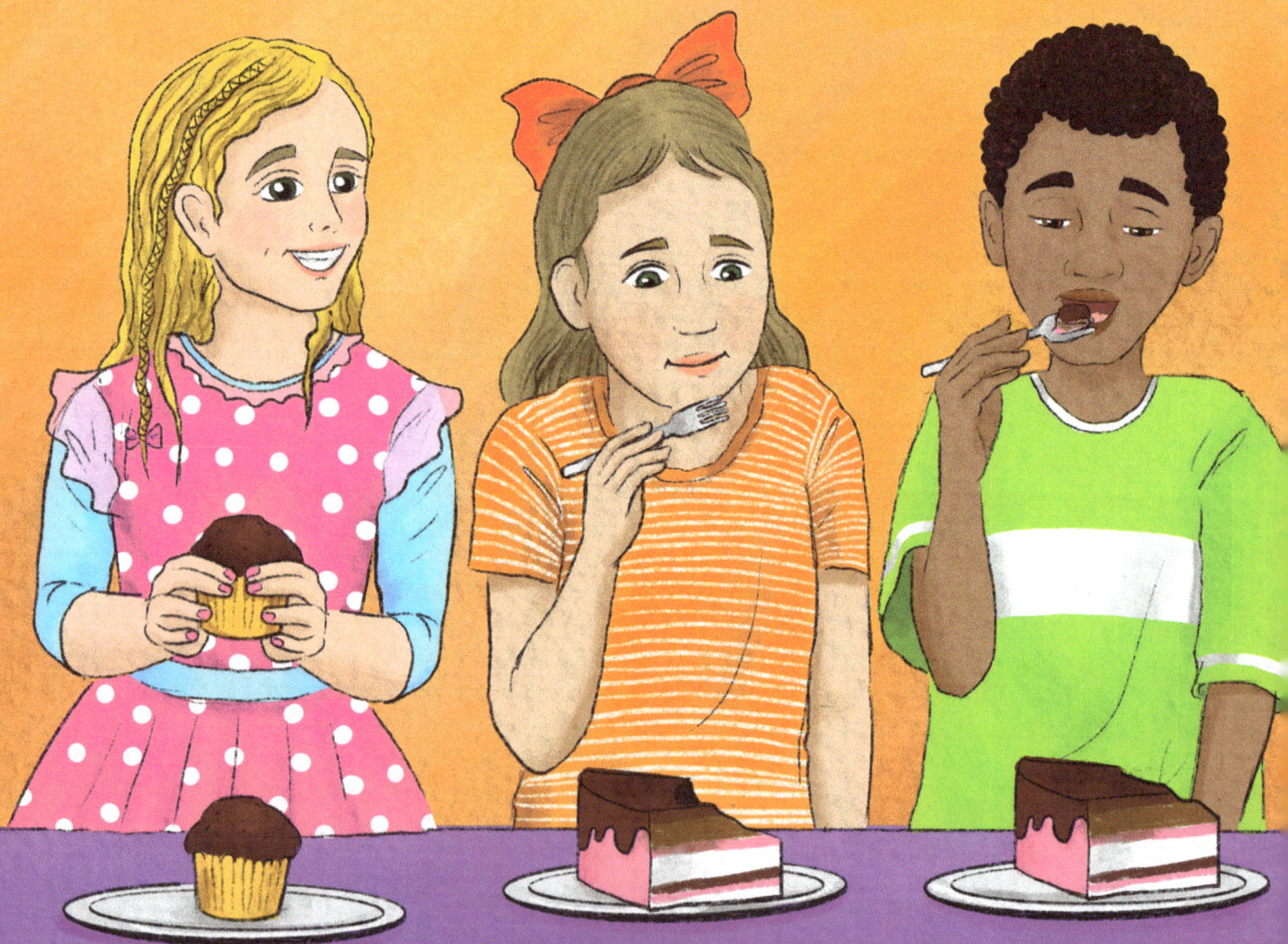

So, Sabina has crafted a simple rule:
Take along your own treats to parties and school.

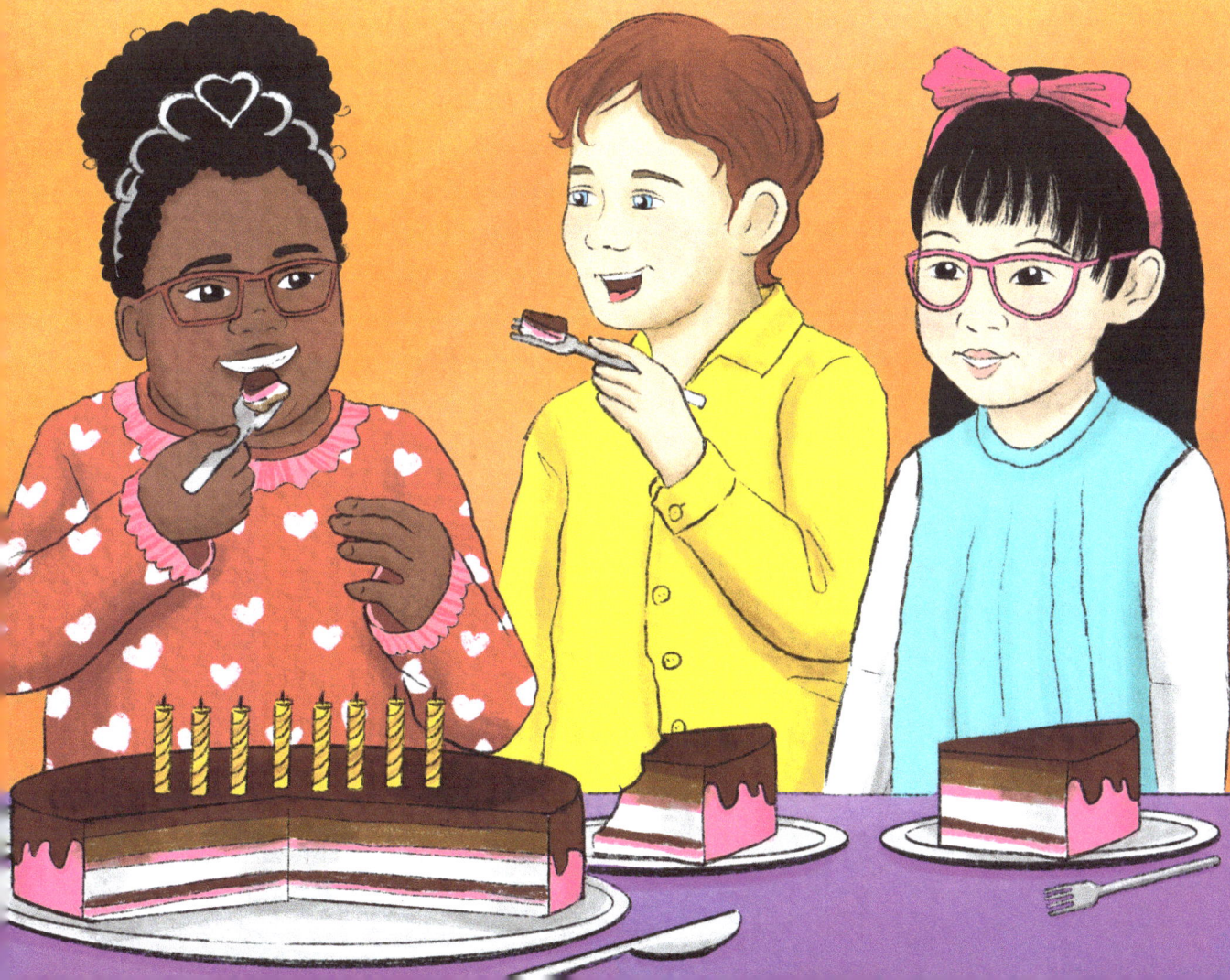

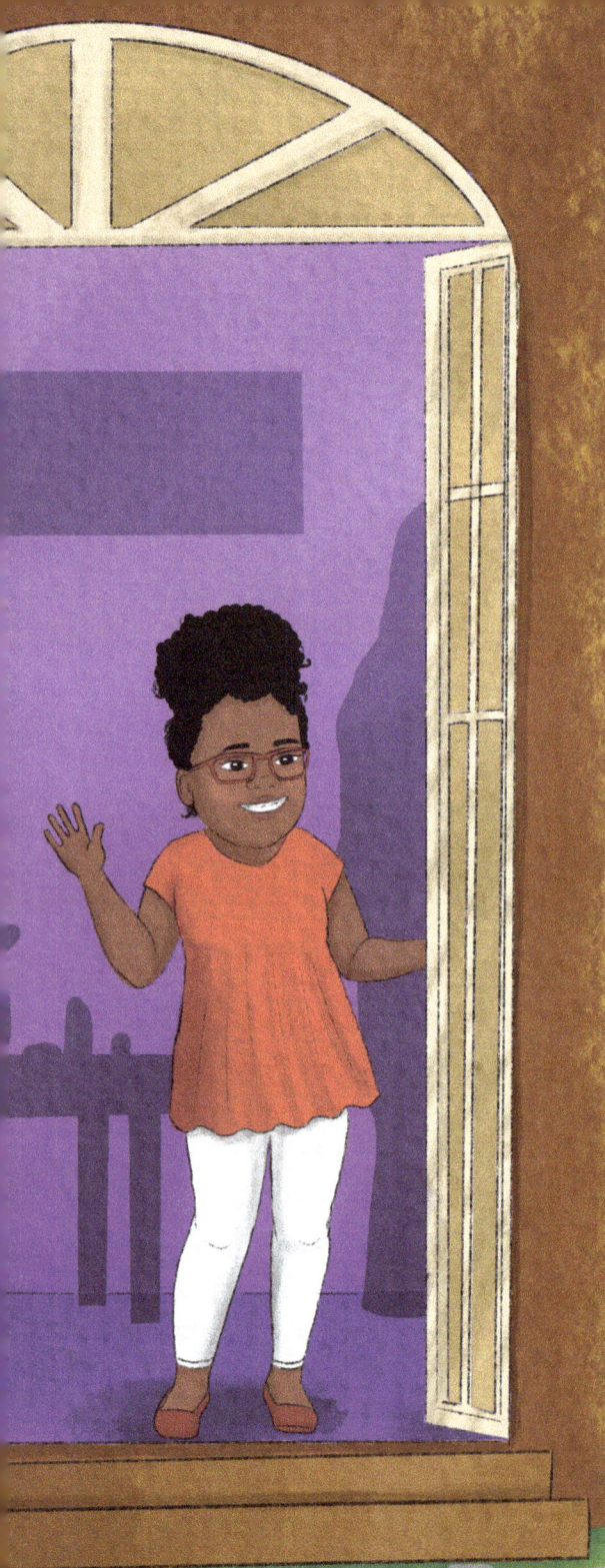

When she visits her friends,
she also packs food

To keep herself safe—
not at all to be rude.

And now that she's used to it,
life is just great.

She's happy and healthy,
and she feels first-rate!

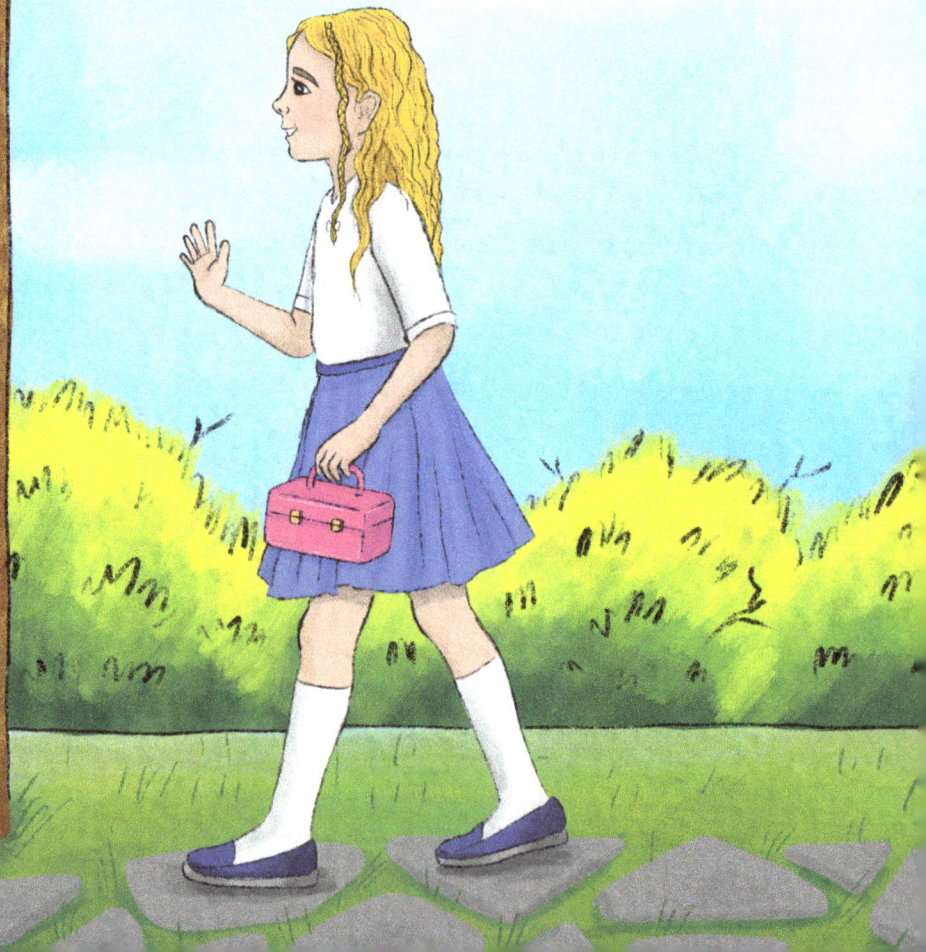

If you can't eat gluten... or nuts... or dairy,
You might think that food can sometimes be scary.
Sabina, though, hopes that this book can help you
Know eating safe foods is possible to do!

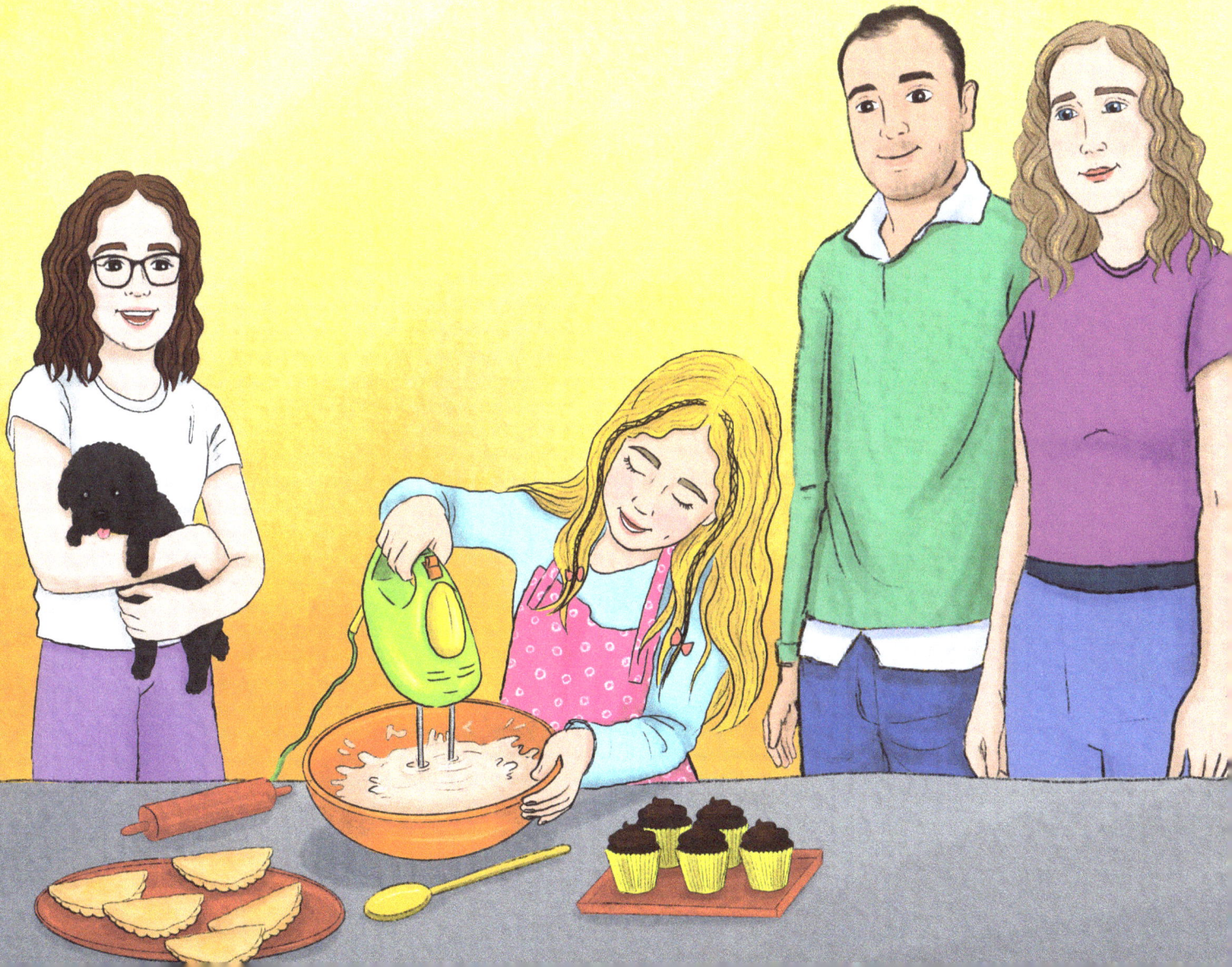

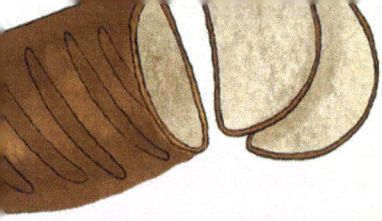

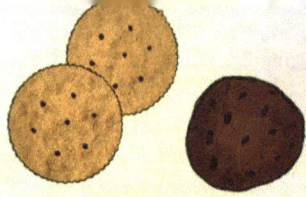

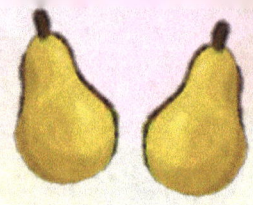

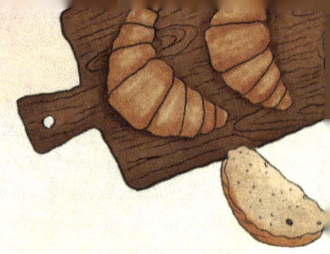

Questions and Answers From the Author
About the Book and Celiac Disease

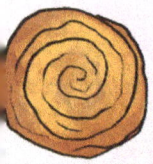

How do you pronounce Sabina? Sabina is pronounced Suh-BEE-nuh.

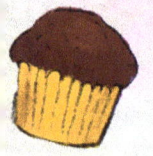

Does Sabina still like to eat dirt and sand? Once Sabina's iron levels were back to normal, she no longer liked the taste of dirt and sand and spit them out right away the next time she tried them. Low iron is a symptom of celiac disease for some people but not others. The same goes for craving dirt and other non-food items—it's a symptom of low iron for some people but not others.

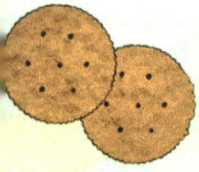

Was it hard to go gluten free? At first it was, and sometimes it still is. Sabina and I (Sabina's mom, the author) were diagnosed with celiac disease during the Covid-19 pandemic while Sabina was engaged in remote learning (attending school virtually on the computer). In a lot of ways, it was an easier time to start eating gluten free because we were trying to keep our family and other families safe from the coronavirus by not getting together in person or going to restaurants, and we could just focus on learning what products to buy, how to prepare gluten-free foods, and how to bake with gluten-free flour. With a little practice, we learned that gluten-free meals and desserts can be just as good or even better than gluten-containing food.

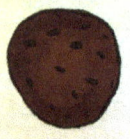

Eating outside the home (traveling, going to restaurants, parties, school, and other people's homes) is the toughest part about having celiac disease, but we've learned that planning ahead makes it much easier!

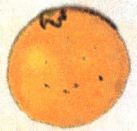

How did you prepare gluten-free meals before you cleaned out your kitchen? For cooking and mixing, we only used our stainless steel pots and pans, stainless steel utensils, and glass and ceramic bowls because they are the easiest materials to clean thoroughly. We still stick to those materials when we stay somewhere with a kitchen while traveling. We also make sure to use a new sponge that never comes into contact with gluten. By the way, you can also do this at home if your kitchen isn't entirely gluten free. Check out nevaryanbooks.com for more shared-kitchen tips.

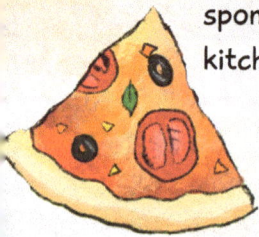

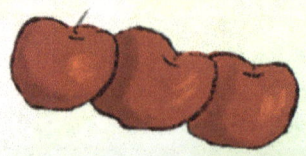

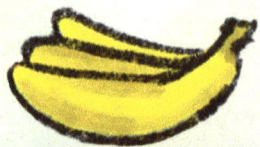

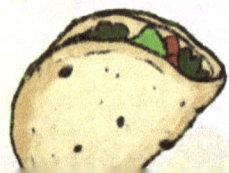

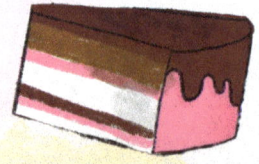

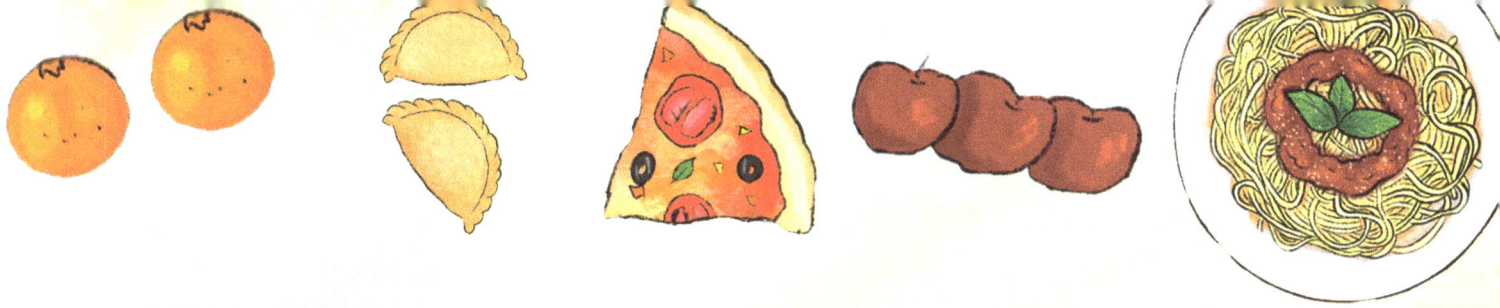

What are the most unexpected places gluten can be hiding? When we first started learning what we could and couldn't eat, we were surprised that Twizzlers, Rice Krispies, Cheerios, and soy sauce all contain gluten. Twizzlers contain wheat flour, Rice Krispies contain malt (which comes from barley), Cheerios, although labeled gluten free in the United States, contain oats that have had cross-contact with gluten, and soy sauce is made with wheat. Luckily, there are gluten-free brands to choose from, so celiacs can eat safe versions of all their favorite foods.

Now we choose very carefully when buying products for our lips (like lip balm and lipstick) and our mouths (like toothpaste) because they could contain gluten. In addition, we always wash our hands before eating. Sometimes we don't even realize we've touched gluten and could end up ingesting it just by having it on our hands! Hand sanitizer kills germs, not gluten, so we make sure to wash with soap and water.

Can you be sure a food, medicine, or other product is gluten free by reading the ingredients on the label? Not always. Even if a product has no gluten in its ingredients, it could have had cross-contact with gluten through processing. Also, ingredients such as malt, "natural flavors," or "smoke flavoring," among others, could be derived from barley, even if barley is not stated on the list of ingredients. Look for a "certified gluten free" statement or logo for the safest food choices. Since not all gluten-free foods and products in the U.S. are labeled gluten free, do internet research or contact the company for more information. If you're not sure, don't eat or use it or give it to anyone who is gluten free.

By the way, there are many countries that do an excellent job of gluten-free labeling. In Argentina (where Sabina has family), there is a national symbol for safe gluten-free foods and products. We really enjoy how easy it is to choose safe foods when we visit there!

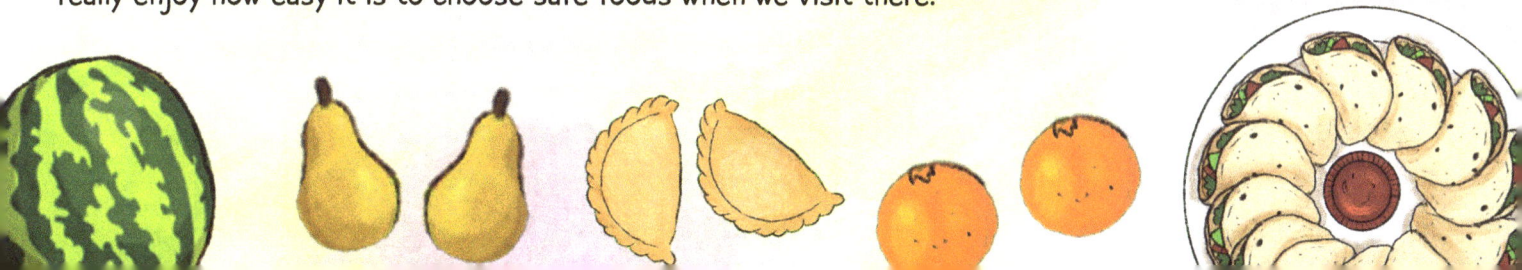

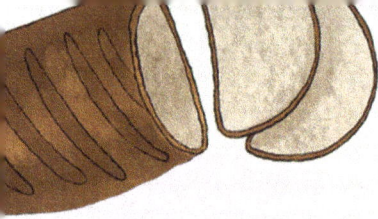

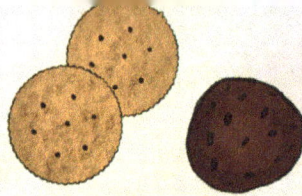

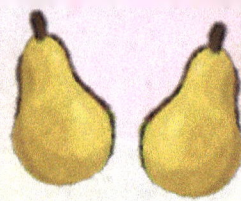

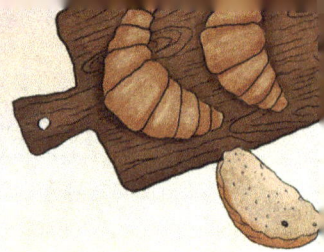

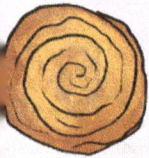

What happens to the body when a person with celiac disease eats gluten? In a person with celiac disease, the body's immune system reacts to gluten by attacking the lining of the small intestine. It can get so damaged that nutrients from food (like iron in Sabina's case) cannot be absorbed properly. This can lead to all kinds of problematic symptoms and eventually other serious health problems. When a person with celiac disease stops eating gluten, the lining of the small intestine can heal and absorb important nutrients again.

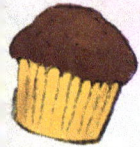

Is there a cure for celiac disease? There is currently no cure or treatment for celiac disease other than following a gluten-free diet, but research is underway all over the world. Maybe someday soon there will be a cure or alternative treatment!

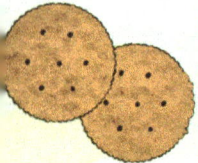

Is it common for people to have celiac disease and not know it? Yes! Even if you're having typical celiac disease symptoms, it's not always the first thing doctors think to check for. If you have ongoing gastrointestinal issues (like vomiting, diarrhea, constipation, or abdominal pain), other unexplained symptoms (like headaches, fatigue, skin issues, inflammation, low iron levels, or slow growth, among others), or if someone in your family has celiac disease, you should ask your doctor to refer you to a gastroenterologist (a GI doctor) to test your blood. It's a very simple first step in diagnosing your symptoms.

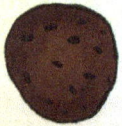

Should you stop eating gluten before getting tested for celiac disease? No! If you plan to get tested for celiac disease, make sure you continue to eat gluten every day before you get your blood tested. Eating gluten free can cause your blood tests to indicate that you don't have celiac disease, even if you actually have it.

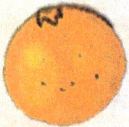

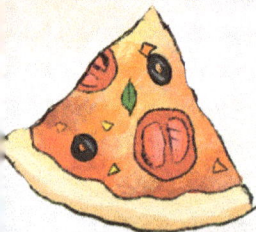

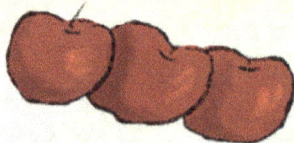

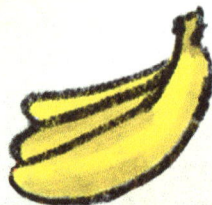

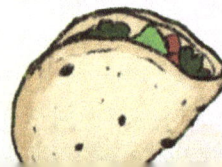

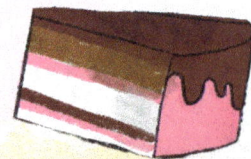

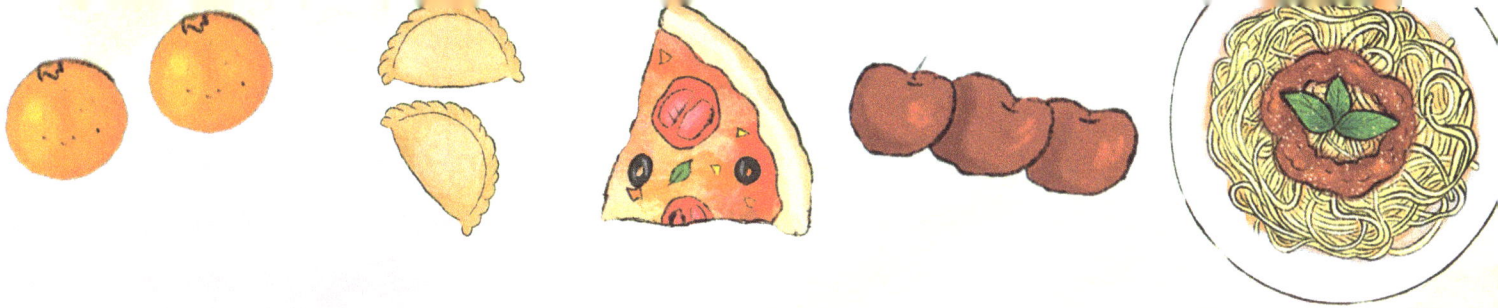

Can you find out if you have celiac disease with just a blood test? Many people (like Sabina's grandma and the author, Sabina's mom) also have an endoscopy and biopsy after their blood is tested if the results point to celiac disease. During an endoscopy and biopsy, a tiny camera is sent down your throat to find out if there is damage to the lining of the small intestine, and some tissue is taken to be studied as well. In Sabina's case, given her conclusive blood test results and her mother's diagnosis of celiac disease, her GI doctor determined she had celiac disease without conducting an endoscopy and biopsy.

What's some good advice for people with celiac disease? Be sure to reach out to other people with celiac disease. There are in-person and online groups for grownups, kids, and families that can help you feel supported and give you lots of helpful tips. Many are run by medical professionals.

In addition to your GI doctor, another medical professional who can be really helpful to you when you're learning how to eat gluten free is a registered dietitian who specializes in celiac disease. Doing careful research through books, articles, podcasts, and online groups can be very useful as well. Check out nevaryanbooks.com for helpful resources!

Is it okay for people who don't have celiac disease to eat gluten free? Yes! Gluten (wheat, barley, or rye) is not essential to a healthy diet. There are other gluten-free whole grains and starchy vegetables that are delicious and healthy for you. So, anyone can eat gluten free and be healthy. Some people who don't have celiac disease but are sensitive to gluten or have gluten intolerance find that they feel much better on a gluten-free diet as well. Can you guess who else in our family eats gluten free? It's our dog! We feed her gluten-free food and treats so we don't have to worry about gluten crumbs or her sweet doggie kisses!

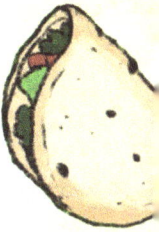

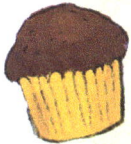

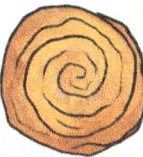

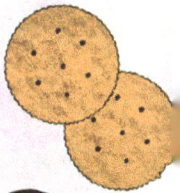

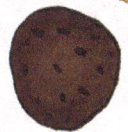

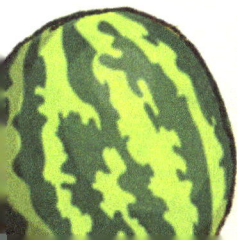

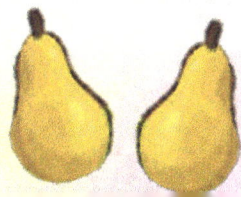

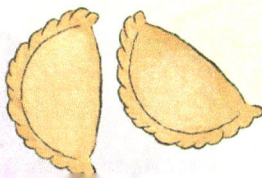

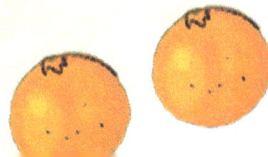

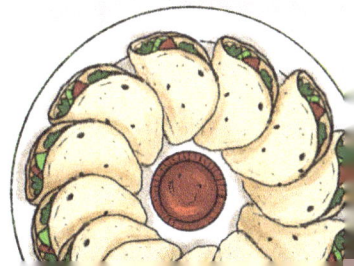

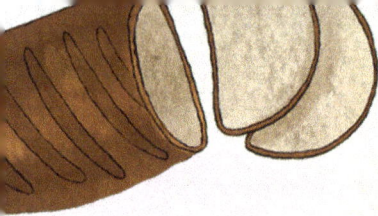

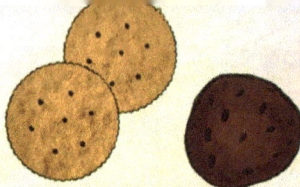

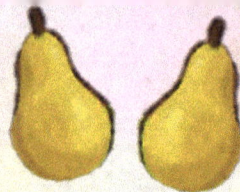

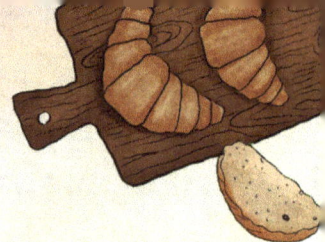

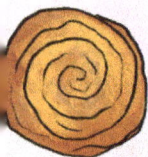

What if you don't have celiac disease? Can you help? Yes! Even if you don't have celiac disease (or gluten sensitivity or intolerance), you now know a lot more about it, and you can be supportive of a friend or family member who might have it.

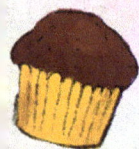

Also, if you live in the United States, you can contact your Senators and Members of Congress and ask them to require barley and rye to be listed on product labels as allergens (along with wheat, which is already required by law to be listed as an allergen). This would clarify whether an ingredient like malt or "natural flavors" is derived from a gluten-containing grain. You can also ask for gluten-free testing and labeling of gluten-free products to be mandatory, not voluntary as is currently the case. Maybe if we all speak up, we can change the laws to make choosing gluten-free products much easier and safer.

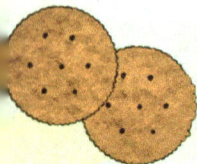

You can even help raise money for celiac disease research. Check out nevaryanbooks.com for a list of organizations doing great work.

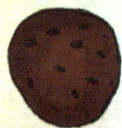

Do you have a question for the author? Click on the "Contact" page of her website (nevaryanbooks.com) and send in your question. It might even be featured in bonus content for readers! Also, check out nevaryanbooks.com for helpful resources about celiac disease and eating gluten free.

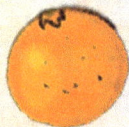

Acknowledgements: I would like to thank Jules Shepard (gfJules) for helping me better understand gluten-free labeling laws in the U.S. I am profoundly grateful for her time and generosity!

I would also like to thank Roslyn Duffy, RD, for her helpful insights and encouragement (and for being a great mom).

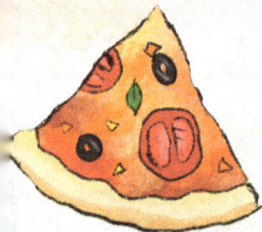

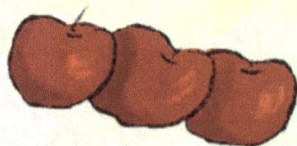

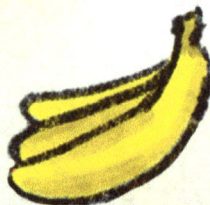

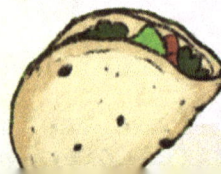

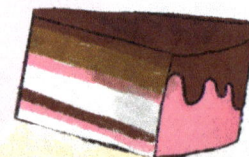

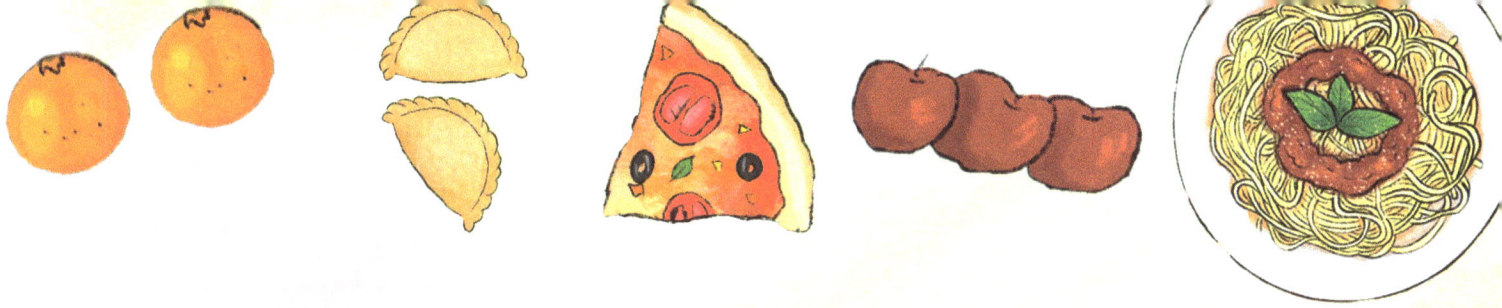

About the Author:

Neva Ryan, author of *The Very Hungry Toilets*, loves writing books for people of all ages, especially children. She is also an educator and translator in Chicago, where she lives with her husband, two daughters, and their little dog. As you know from the book, she has celiac disease and wrote this book about her daughter's celiac journey to help kids and grownups learn all about it.

Check out nevaryanbooks.com to find her other books as well as helpful resources on celiac disease and eating gluten free!

About the Illustrator:

Behnaz Hajielyasi is an illustrator and graphic designer who specializes in creating lovable children's book characters as well as vector graphics, web pages, logos, and more. She lives in Germany with her husband.

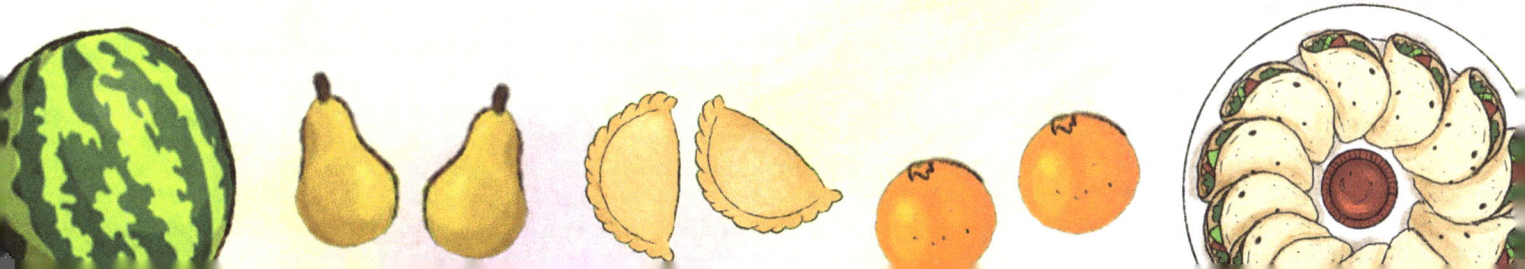

www.ingramcontent.com/pod-product-compliance
Lightning Source LLC
Chambersburg PA
CBHW042344030426
42335CB00030B/3453